THE VACCINE DEBATE

Recent Titles in Health and Medical Issues Today

THE VACCINE DEBATE

Tish Davidson

Health and Medical Issues Today

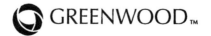

GREENWOOD™

An Imprint of ABC-CLIO, LLC
Santa Barbara, California • Denver, Colorado

Library of Congress Cataloging-in-Publication Data

Names: Davidson, Tish, author.
Title: The vaccine debate / Tish Davidson.
Description: Santa Barbara, California : Greenwood, [2019] | Series: Health and
    medical issues today | Includes bibliographical references and index.
Identifiers: LCCN 2018030122 (print) | LCCN 2018031675 (ebook) |
    ISBN 9781440843549 (ebook) | ISBN 9781440843532 (print : alk. paper)
Subjects: | MESH: Vaccines | Vaccination | Treatment Outcome | Public Opinion |
    Mandatory Programs—ethics
Classification: LCC QR189 (ebook) | LCC QR189 (print) | NLM QW 805 |
    DDC 615.3/72—dc23
LC record available at https://lccn.loc.gov/2018030122

ISBN: 978-1-4408-4353-2 (print)
      978-1-4408-4354-9 (ebook)

23 22 21 20 19   1 2 3 4 5

This book is also available as an eBook.

Greenwood
An Imprint of ABC-CLIO, LLC

ABC-CLIO, LLC
147 Castilian Drive
Santa Barbara, CA 93117
www.abc-clio.com

This book is printed on acid-free paper ∞

Manufactured in the United States of America

In memory of my father, Paul M. Stouffer, musician and composer

CONTENTS

SERIES FOREWORD

Every day, the public is bombarded with information on developments in medicine and health care. Whether it is on the latest techniques in treatment or research or on concerns over public health threats, this information directly affects the lives of people more than almost any other issue. Although there are many sources for understanding these topics—from websites and blogs to newspapers and magazines—students and ordinary citizens often need one resource that makes sense of the complex health and medical issues affecting their daily lives.

The *Health and Medical Issues Today* series provides just such a one-stop resource for obtaining a solid overview of the most controversial areas of health care in the 21st century. Each volume addresses one topic and provides a balanced summary of what is known. These volumes provide an excellent first step for students and lay people interested in understanding how health care works in our society today.

Each volume is broken into several parts to provide readers and researchers with easy access to the information they need:

Part I provides overview chapters on background information—including chapters on such areas as the historical, scientific, medical, social, and legal issues involved—that a citizen needs to intelligently understand the topic.

Part II provides capsule examinations of the most heated contemporary issues and debates, and analyzes in a balanced manner the viewpoints held by various advocates in the debates.

Part III provides case studies that show examples of the concepts discussed in the previous parts.

A selection of reference material, such as a timeline of important events, a directory of organizations, and a bibliography, serve as the best next step in learning about the topic at hand.

The *Health and Medical Issues Today* series strives to provide readers with all the information needed to begin making sense of some of the most important debates going on in the world today. The series includes volumes on such topics as stem cell research, obesity, gene therapy, alternative medicine, organ transplantation, mental health, and more.

PREFACE

Vaccines save lives. They have eradicated the scourge of smallpox, a disease that over the centuries killed millions and left millions more disabled. They are on the verge of eradicating polio and have prevented thousands of deaths from diphtheria and birth defects from rubella (German measles) infection. Yet, despite very clear evidence that vaccines save lives and prevent disabilities, there has always been some opposition to their use. The strength of this opposition has varied both geographically and across time.

Until the middle of the 20th century, most people had personal experience with some vaccine-preventable diseases such as diphtheria, polio, tetanus, and measles. They understood the damage these diseases could cause and welcomed the opportunity to avoid illness through immunization. Opposition to vaccination was minimal.

As dreaded diseases declined in developed countries and awareness of their risks faded, some people began questioning the safety of vaccines and the need for vaccination. The medical community responded with statistics demonstrating that vaccines have a high rate of effectiveness and low rate of serious side effects. It warned that outbreaks of vaccine-preventable diseases were inevitable unless a large percentage of the population was vaccinated. Although this satisfied most people, some remained opposed to vaccination.

The uncensored platform of the internet in the 21st century has substantially increased the scope and intensity of the debate about the safety and value of vaccine. Still, most parents consider vaccination a positive health intervention. Vaccination rates across the 50 states in the United States range from 99 percent in Mississippi and Maryland to 87 percent in

Colorado. But despite data showing vaccines are safe and effective, a substantial number of parents, if not outright vaccine rejectors, choose to skip certain vaccinations or insist on modifying the medically recommended vaccination schedule for their children.

This book considers both sides of the vaccine debate. Part I explains how vaccines work, the diseases they prevent, and the way vaccines are tested, manufactured, and regulated. Part II considers some of the factors that influence individual vaccination decisions. This is followed by an analysis of six specific areas of controversy by examining the anti-vaccinationist view and the medical establishment's view of the topic. Part III illustrates some of the consequences of vaccine choices individual parents made. It is hoped that readers will approach this material thoughtfully, keeping in mind the reliability of the sources of information presented when considering the validity of the viewpoints of each side.

ACKNOWLEDGMENTS

If it takes a village to raise a child, it takes a team to birth a book. Although there is only one name on the cover, many people nurtured this manuscript. Thanks and appreciation are owed to my outstanding editor Maxine Taylor and the production staff at ABC-CLIO and Apex CoVantage for their patience and attention to detail. Thanks also to the Thursday Night Writers, Evelyn LaTorre, Jan Salinas, and Joyce Cortez, for hunting down murky explanations and making them more lucid. Finally, without the support of my family and their tolerance for my "vaccine sermons," this book would not have happened.

PART I

Overview and Background Information

CHAPTER 1

Vaccines and Health

Ask a random selection of parents whether their children have been vaccinated and you get a lot of different answers.

"Of course, my child is vaccinated. Vaccines save lives," one parent will tell you. "It would be crazy not to vaccinate."

"Vaccines harm innocent children and cause lifelong developmental problems. Why would I put my child at risk by vaccinating?" asks another.

"The law says my child must be vaccinated to attend school, so I obey the law," says the third.

"My child, my decision," exclaims the fourth. "The government should not force a medical procedure on my child against my wishes."

What is the big deal about vaccines? For one thing, they are given to healthy children to prevent them from getting sick, not to cure a disease that they already have. The diseases vaccines prevent, although dangerous, are often rare or unfamiliar. Many people also find the way vaccines work strange and hard to grasp. Why would a vaccine containing part of an organism that causes a disease protect children from that same disease? Finally, compulsory vaccination laws favor community health over individual choice. Parents are asked to trust their government and have faith that the pharmaceutical industry is putting the well-being of their children above profits. Mix the intense protective emotions parents feel toward their children with these various points of view and you have the great vaccine debate.

WHAT ARE VACCINES?

A vaccine is a biological preparation that, when introduced into the body, creates long-term protection against contracting a specific disease.

The World Health Organization (WHO) claims: "The impact of vaccination on the health of the world's peoples is hard to exaggerate. With the exception of safe water, nothing else, not even antibiotics, has had such a major effect on the reduction of mortality [deaths] and morbidity [illness and disability] and on population growth." The WHO estimates immunization against only four diseases—diphtheria, tetanus, pertussis (whooping cough), and measles—prevents 2 to 3 million deaths worldwide each year and that an additional 1.5 million deaths could be prevented annually using vaccines already developed if access to these vaccines were expanded.

The greatest success for a vaccine occurred in 1980 when smallpox was declared eradicated after an extended international immunization program. Before eradication, smallpox killed as many as one-third of the people it infected and left many survivors disabled or disfigured. Between 1880 and 1980, an estimated half billion people died of the disease. The United States declared routine vaccination against smallpox unnecessary in 1972.

Poliomyelitis is now the second human disease likely to be eradicated worldwide. The last case polio originating in the United States occurred in 1979. In the first half of 2018, Afghanistan reported 10 cases of wild polio and Pakistan 3 cases. The Democratic Republic of Congo, Somalia, and Nigeria reported a total of 14 cases of vaccine-derived polio. Syria reported no cases but remained on a watch list because of cases reported in 2017. The U.S. Centers for Disease Control and Prevention (CDC) still recommends polio vaccinations for children because the disease can be brought into the country by travelers from places where it still exists. Many vaccine-skeptic parents in developed countries dispute the necessity of this vaccine because the disease is rare.

IMMUNE SYSTEM BASICS

To better grasp how vaccines work and why they cause controversy, it is necessary to understand some basic immune system vocabulary. The immune system is the body's defense against disease-causing viruses, bacteria, fungi, and parasites, collectively known as pathogens. These pathogens have protein molecules on their surface called antigens. The word "antigen" comes from a combination of the words "*anti*body" and "*gener*ator." Any foreign material that stimulates the immune system to produce antibodies is an antigen.

Antibodies are tiny Y-shaped proteins produced by specialized immune system cells called plasma cells. They are 10 times smaller than viruses and 200 times smaller than bacteria. Once the antibody-generating system is cranked up, plasma cells can produce 120,000 identical antibodies per minute for three to five days. These antibodies flood the bloodstream where they seek out and bind with antigens on the surface of a single, specific pathogen. Once the antigen and the antibody bind, the pathogen is inactivated. Thus, pathogens make us sick, and antibodies help us to recover.

There is, however, a drawback to the system of antibody generation. The first time the immune system meets a new pathogen, it takes about two weeks for plasma cells to begin functioning. During this two-week period, a person develops symptoms of illness. Sometimes diseases become destructive so rapidly (e.g., Ebola virus disease or anthrax) that the individual dies before enough antibodies are produced to stop the pathogen. This slow response to the first encounter with a pathogen is called the primary response.

Making antibodies is only one part of the primary response. If the individual survives, the immune system also creates memory cells that "remember" the pathogen. If the exact same pathogen later invades the body, memory cells immediately kick the antibody-generating process into high gear. Within about three days, the immune system creates a huge number of antibodies against the pathogen. This quick production of antibodies on subsequent encounters with a pathogen for which the immune system has made memory cells is called the secondary response. In a secondary response, antibodies destroy the pathogen fast enough that the individual does not get sick. When an individual has made memory cells against a disease, this person has developed immunity to that disease. Immunity acquired from having the disease and recovering is called active natural immunity.

VACCINES AND THE IMMUNE SYSTEM

The value of vaccines is that they allow an individual to develop immunity to a disease without first contracting the disease and becoming sick. The key to this outcome is the presence of modified pathogen antigens in the vaccine. Some vaccines contain killed or inactivated versions of the pathogen itself. Others are genetically engineered so that only antigens from the pathogen and not the whole pathogen are used. Chapter 3 gives more details on how vaccines are created.

What all vaccines have in common is that the antigens must either be weakened enough or be in a partial form so that they cannot cause the disease they are immunizing against. On the other hand, they must be strong enough to stimulate the production of antibodies and the development of memory cells. When this balance is achieved, the individual acquires immunity without risking the health effects of having the disease and without becoming contagious and passing the disease to others in the community. Immunity acquired through vaccination is called artificially acquired active immunity.

Naturally acquired immunity, created by having a disease and recovering, is the strongest form of immunity, but the individual experiences all the symptoms and risks associated with having the disease. The strength of artificial immunity created by vaccination can last a lifetime or for a shorter period, depending on the disease, the effectiveness of the vaccine, and the strength of the individual's immune system response. The process of developing immunity involves a long chain of cellular events that will be discussed in Chapter 2.

VACCINE-PREVENTABLE DISEASES

As of 2018, vaccines can prevent at least 33 human diseases. Twenty of these diseases are caused by viruses, 11 by bacteria, and 2 by bacterial toxins, which are damaging waste products produced by some bacteria. Seventeen vaccines are routinely used in the United States, while another nine are available to travelers visiting countries where the disease is prevalent, select military members, or people whose jobs put them at high risk for contracting a particular disease (e.g., workers in vaccine manufacturing, veterinarians, aid workers after a natural disaster). At least eight additional vaccines are used in other countries but are not licensed for use in the United States.

Vaccines in use as of 2018 are listed in Table 1.1. These vaccines, the diseases they prevent, and their potential side effects are discussed in more

Table 1.1 Vaccine-Preventable Diseases

Vaccines Used in the United States	Organism Vaccine Protects Against	Target Population for First Dose[†]
Adenovirus	Type 4 and type 7 adenovirus that cause respiratory illnesses similar to influenza	Approved for military members; ages 17–50 years only
Anthrax	*Bacillus anthracis* bacterium that can cause fever, shock, inflammation of brain	Most military members and overseas defense contractors; some people who handle wool, meat, and hides; ages 18–65 years
Cholera	*Vibrio cholerae* bacterium that causes diarrhea, vomiting, dehydration	Not routinely used in United States; may be given to adults traveling to areas where cholera is prevalent; limited effectiveness

Vaccines Used in the United States	Organism Vaccine Protects Against	Target Population for First Dose[†]
Diphtheria	Toxin of the bacterium *Corynebacterium diphtheriae* that causes a covering to form at the back of the throat creating breathing problems	Children starting age 2 months
Hepatitis A	Hepatitis A virus that can cause permanent liver damage	Children between 12 and 23 months; travelers to Mexico, Central and South America, Africa, Asia, and Eastern Europe; men who have sex with men; people who use injectable street drugs
Hepatitis B	Hepatitis B virus that can cause permanent liver damage and liver cancer	Newborns; men who have sex with men; people who use injectable street drugs
Haemophilus influenzae type b (Hib)	*Haemophilus influenzae* type b that causes bacterial meningitis	Children age 2 months
Human papillomavirus (HPV)	Multiple types of HPV that cause genital warts and cervical, penile, and anal cancer	Girls and boys starting between ages 9 and 11 years
Influenza	Three or four strains of influenza virus that cause fever and secondary pneumonia. Composition of vaccine changes annually	Every year for everyone over age 6 months
Japanese encephalitis	Japanese encephalitis *Flavirus* that causes fever, seizures, coma	Travelers over age 2 months spending one month or more in rural Asia where the disease is common
Measles (rubeola)	*Morbillivirus* that causes fever, and can cause seizures, brain damage	Children age 12 months
Meningococcal disease	Multiple types of *Neisseria meningitidis* bacteria that cause meningitis	11–12 years
Mumps	*Rubulavirus* that causes fever, swollen glands, and possible meningitis, deafness, sterility	Children ages 12 months
Pertussis (whooping cough)	*Bordetella pertussis* bacterium that causes severe coughing, difficulty breathing, seizures	Children age 2 months

(Continued)

Table 1.1 (Continued)

Vaccines Used in the United States	Organism Vaccine Protects Against	Target Population for First Dose[†]
Pneumococcal disease	Multiple types of *Streptococcus pneumoniae* bacteria that cause pneumonia	Children age 2 months and adults age 65 and older
Poliomyelitis (inactivated vaccine)	*Poliovirus* that causes paralysis	Children age 2 months
Rabies	*Lyssavirus* that causes death by attacking the nervous system	Only people likely to be exposed to rabid animals (pre-exposure vaccination) or who have been bitten by a potentially rabid animal (postexposure vaccination); no age restrictions
Rotavirus	*Rotavirus* that causes severe diarrhea and dehydration in infants	Children age 2 months
Rubella (German measles)	*Rubella* virus that can cause severe birth defects in fetus	Children age 12 months
Shingles	*Varicella zoster* virus. Same as chickenpox virus, but in older adults causes fever, painful blisters, nerve pain	Adults over age 50 years
Smallpox	*Variola major* and *Variola minor* viruses that cause fever, painful rash, high mortality	Some military members because of the threat of bioterrorism; no age restrictions
Tetanus (lockjaw)	Toxin of the bacterium *Clostridium tetani* that causes severe muscle contraction that can interfere with eating and breathing	Children age 2 months with a booster shot every 10 years for adolescents and adults (pre-exposure vaccination) and all ages after certain types of bites or wounds (postexposure vaccination)
Tuberculosis (Bacille Calmette-Guérin vaccine)	*Mycobacterium tuberculosis* bacterium that causes lung disease	Newborns and infants in developing countries where the disease is common; legal but rarely used in the United States; also used to treat noninvasive bladder cancer in adults
Typhoid fever (enteric fever)	Various types of *Salmonella enterica* bacteria that cause high fever, delirium, gastrointestinal damage	Travelers where the disease is common, mainly underdeveloped countries; 80 percent of cases come from Bangladesh, China, India, Indonesia, Laos, Nepal, Pakistan, or Vietnam

Vaccines Used in the United States	Organism Vaccine Protects Against	Target Population for First Dose[†]
Varicella (Chickenpox)	*Varicella zoster* virus that causes rash, itching, fever	Children age 12 months
Yellow fever	*Flavivirus* that causes bleeding from multiple sites, organ failure	Travelers to Africa, South America, and some Caribbean islands

Vaccines Not Available in the United States		
Dengue	*Flavivirus* that causes fever and intense muscle and joint pain	Not licensed in United States; as of 2018, licensed in many tropical and subtropical countries
Ebola virus disease	*Ebolavirus* that causes vomiting, bleeding from mucous membranes, headaches, muscle aches, tissue swelling, low blood pressure, fever, death	Limited supply available; not formally licensed but available for use on an emergency basis; licensure expected in 2018
Kyasanur Forest disease	*Flavivirus* that causes fever, internal and external bleeding, death	Not licensed for use in the United States; disease and vaccine use are limited to the west coast of India
Leptospirosis	*Leptospira interrogans*, a spirochete bacterium that causes meningitis, hepatitis, nephritis, death	Not licensed for use in the United States; available in China, Cuba, Japan, and France; limited effectiveness
Plague	*Yersinia pestis* bacterium that causes flu-like symptoms, swollen lymph nodes, 30–60% fatalities	No longer available in the United States and little used elsewhere due to limited effectiveness and ability to tread disease with antibiotics
Poliomyelitis (oral polio vaccine)	*Poliovirus* that causes paralysis	Used in many developing countries because of ease of administration; highly effective
Q fever	*Coxiella burnetii* bacterium that causes high fever, headache, cough, gastrointestinal symptoms	Not licensed for use in the United States; available in Australia, Canada, and elsewhere for high-risk populations
Tickborne encephalitis	*Flavivirus* that causes brain inflammation	Not licensed for use in the United States; commonly used in Europe and Asia

[†]Recommendations based on information from the U.S. Centers for Disease Control and Prevention, 2018 for healthy Americans. Recommendations in other countries and for specific subpopulations with compromised health will vary. Many vaccines require multiple doses to establish and maintain immunity.

detail in Chapter 5. Many vaccines come in more than one formulation and require more than one dose to stimulate adequate immunity. Table 1.1 indicates only the earliest age at which the first dose of vaccine is recommended in the United States as of 2018.

VACCINES AND SOCIETY

Vaccine-preventable diseases are serious illnesses with the potential to cause permanent damage or death. Over the past 100 years, large-scale vaccination programs have greatly reduced the number of people who become infected with these diseases. For example, in the mid-1920s, before an effective diphtheria vaccine was widely available, at least 200,000 people in the United States contracted diphtheria every year. Between 5 percent and 10 percent died, with the death rate rising to 20 percent in children younger than five years. However, after almost 100 years of vaccination against diphtheria, no cases are reported in the United States in most years and only a handful of cases occur in Europe.

Polio caused 57,879 cases of paralysis and 3,145 deaths in the United States in 1952. A vaccine against polio was licensed in 1955. By 1965, after only 10 years of polio immunizations, the number of paralytic polio cases had dropped to 61 with only 16 deaths. Cases of measles, mumps, rubella (German measles), and *Haemophilus Influenzae* type b (Hib) have all shown 99 percent decreases since vaccines against these diseases came into use. Despite this, anti-vaccination parents challenge the safety and effectiveness of vaccination.

Public Health Benefits

In addition to creating improved resistance to disease in individuals who are immunized, vaccines provide public health benefits in several ways.

- When enough people in a community are vaccinated against a disease, the pathogen finds it more difficult to pass successfully from person to person. This protects the entire community against widespread outbreaks of the disease, a condition called herd immunity. Normally, about 93 percent of individuals must have immunity to a pathogen to prevent an epidemic (see Chapter 2, Herd Immunity).
- Vaccination of healthy individuals helps protect people who cannot safely receive specific vaccines for medical reasons. A disease such as chickenpox that is often mild in healthy individuals can be fatal to people with compromised immune systems such as those receiving

chemotherapy, individuals who have inherited immune system deficiencies (there are about 250 of these disorders), and people with diseases that attack immune system cells. The most common of these immune-attacking diseases is HIV/AIDS.

- Contracting a vaccine-preventable illness results in increased doctor visits and may require hospitalization, especially among the very young and the elderly. Because vaccines prevent pain, suffering, and disability from complications, health care and rehabilitation costs are reduced, as are days lost from work. Even if a vaccine is not 100 percent effective, it can reduce the severity of a disease.

Vaccination of Animals

The successful eradication of smallpox and near eradication of polio through vaccination are possible because the viruses that cause these diseases infect only humans. However, many pathogens infect both humans and animals. Diseases that can be transmitted from animals to humans are called zoonoses. Many vaccine-preventable diseases are zoonotic. Infected animals serve as a reservoir for the disease and create a path for continuing infection in humans either by direct contact or through vectors such as infected mosquitoes, ticks, or fleas.

Vigorous animal vaccination programs can prevent millions of people from becoming sick but cannot eradicate a human disease for which there is an animal reservoir. For example, rabies can be passed from animals to humans by the bite of an infected animal. Although the WHO estimates that worldwide 50,000 people die from rabies each year, the disease is rare in the developed world (only 55 cases in the United States since 1990) because of laws requiring dogs and cats to be vaccinated against rabies and programs to put rabies vaccine in bait for wildlife such as raccoons and foxes that are susceptible to the virus.

Brucellosis is a less familiar zoonotic disease of cattle, sheep, and goats. People acquire brucellosis by drinking unpasteurized milk from infected animals. In humans, the disease goes by the names Mediterranean fever, Malta fever, or ungulate fever. It causes fever, headache, joint pain, loss of appetite, weight loss, fatigue, and depression. Mass livestock vaccination has improved herd health and practically eliminated the disease in humans in the United States.

Venezuelan equine encephalitis is a zoonotic disease found in the Caribbean and northern South America. It causes serious to fatal illness in horses, donkeys, and mules. Mosquitoes bite infected animals, become infected, and then pass the disease to humans whom they bite. It takes only

10–100 virus particles to make a person sick. Many people develop only influenza-like symptoms and exhaustion, but up to one-third of infected children go on to develop encephalitis (brain infection), nervous system complications, or death. There is an effective equine vaccine, but none for humans. However, by vaccinating horses and applying mosquito abatement measures, disease outbreaks in humans can be controlled.

Vaccines and Bioterrorism

Vaccines play an ongoing role in defense against bioterrorism. Biological warfare is almost as old as war itself. As early as 300 BCE, the Greeks dumped animal corpses in the wells of their enemies to poison the water supply. The Tartars used catapults to send plague-infected bodies over the walls of the city of Caffa (now Feodosija, Ukraine) during a siege in 1346. Some historians believe this was the source of the Black Death, a form of plague that swept across Europe between 1346 and 1353 killing as many as 200 million people.

In the 20th century, the Japanese practiced biological warfare when they dropped bombs containing 15 million plague-infected fleas on the Chinese cities of Quxian and Ninghsien. This resulted in the death of at least 120 people. More recently, one week after the September 11, 2001, attack on the World Trade Center and the Pentagon in the United States, letters containing powdered anthrax were sent to two U.S. senators and several media outlets. Twenty-two people were infected and five died. The letters were later traced to a disgruntled anthrax researcher who committed suicide before he could be arrested.

Increased concern about acts of terrorism in the 21st century has stimulated research to develop vaccines against biological agents most likely to be capable of quickly killing or sickening many people. These agents include *Bacillus anthracis* (anthrax); *Yersinia pestis* (plague); *Francisella tularensis* (tularemia, a disease that causes high fever, lymph node swelling, chest pain, and difficulty breathing); the viruses that cause hemorrhagic fever (Ebola, Marburg, Lassa, and Machupo); the variola virus (smallpox); toxin from *Clostridium botulinum* (botulism); pathogens that cause Q fever, brucellosis, and typhus; and pathogens that cause disease by contaminating food (e.g., *Salmonella, Shigella*) or water (e.g., *Vibrio cholerae*).

As of 2018, vaccines are available against anthrax, smallpox, Q fever, and cholera. A vaccine exists against plague, but it is not very effective, and the supply of Ebola vaccine is limited. Although smallpox has been eradicated worldwide, the United States and Russia have kept a small amount of smallpox virus frozen in highly secured laboratories for research purposes. Keeping this stock of virus is controversial because there is a small chance that virus could be obtained and used by terrorists as a weapon. For this reason, smallpox vaccine is still made in the United States, and some military members are still vaccinated against the disease.

Recognizing the seriousness of a biological attack or pandemic outbreak of disease, the CDC maintains large quantities medicines and medical supplies, including vaccines, needed to respond to such an event. The program, known as the Strategic National Stockpile (SNS), consists of secret warehouses located at various places so that aid can be delivered to any place in the United States within 12–36 hours. Many aspects of the SNS, such as the warehouse locations, are classified. Nevertheless, it is public knowledge that the SNS contains several hundred thousand doses of smallpox vaccine as well anthrax vaccine and postexposure therapeutic drugs such as antibiotics that could be used to treat plague and other bacterial pathogens. In the event of an emergency, these supplies would be distributed free to all individuals at risk. The need to continually replace vaccines in the SNS as they pass their expiration dates creates significant cost for the federal government. However, it also provides pharmaceutical companies with incentives to research vaccines against pathogens that are potential biological weapons.

VACCINES REMAIN CONTROVERSIAL

Despite the success of vaccination programs in reducing disease and improving public health, a substantial number of people challenge the value of immunization in the United States, United Kingdom, France, Australia, Italy, Japan, and other developed countries. The anti-vaccination movement encompasses people from a range of backgrounds, political orientations, and education levels who have differing objections to vaccines. However, two basic beliefs are shared by anti-vaccinationists. First is the idea that vaccines administered in accordance with government-recommended vaccination schedules have the potential to cause serious harm, especially to children. Second is the anti-vaccinationists' conviction that vaccination should be a personal choice and that they, not the government, should decide if and when to vaccinate.

Beyond these two fundamental beliefs, anti-vaccinationists take variety of positions on what they believe is best for themselves and their children. A small number of strict anti-vaccinationists reject the use of all vaccines. More common are vaccine-skeptic parents. These anti-vaccinationists reject specific vaccines as being either unnecessary (e.g., polio, chickenpox)

or too risky (e.g., measles), but allow their children to receive a few vaccines that they consider essential and low risk.

Vaccine-skeptic and vaccine-hesitant parents also object to the government-
recommended timing for vaccine administration and the use of combination vaccines such as the single shot that immunizes against mumps,
measles, rubella, and chickenpox. These individuals see potential harm
in inoculating children with too many antigens at too young an age. Their
solution is to extend the period between administration of what they decide
are essential vaccines and to delay or skip the administration of others.
Some vaccine-skeptic physicians have developed alternative vaccination
schedules to meet the needs anti-vaccinationist parents while the traditional medical establishment sees this practice as extending the period of
vulnerability for children (see Chapter 11).

Effects of the Vaccine Debate

Despite the widespread acceptance that vaccination results in both personal and public health benefits, a significant percentage of children do not
get all the CDC-recommended vaccines at the recommended times. Some
of these children have medical conditions that prevent vaccination. Others have economic and logistical barriers to receiving routine health care.
Many, however, are healthy children whose parents have sought exemptions from vaccinations for nonmedical reasons. Vaccination requirements
and permissible exemptions vary considerably from state to state.

The following list shows the percentage of children ages 19–35 months
who have not received the recommended doses of specific vaccines the
CDC has determined are appropriate for their age. The data are from 2017.
They give an approximate idea of the extent of the vaccine skepticism in
the United States and the degree to which vaccines are viewed as either
potentially harmful or unnecessary.

- Diphtheria, tetanus, pertussis (DTP, DT, or DTaP): 15.4% incom-
  pletely vaccinated
- Polio: 6.3%
- Measles, mumps, rubella (MMR): 8.1%
- *Haemophilus influenzae* type b (Hib): 17.3%
- Hepatitis B (Hep B): 8.1%
- Chickenpox (varicella): 8.2%
- Pneumococcal conjugate vaccine: 15.9%
- All age-appropriate doses of the combined seven-vaccine series
  listed above (i.e., not fully vaccinated): 27.8%

To review, vaccines are biological preparations that contain antigens that stimulate the body to make antibodies against a specific disease. The creation of antibodies and long-lived memory cells is the key to creating immunity. Immunity, whether naturally acquired by disease or artificially acquired by immunization, prevents individuals from becoming sick if they encounter the pathogen that causes a disease against which they have created memory cells. Even when vaccines are not 100 percent effective, they create partial immunity that reduces symptoms and severity of the disease.

As of 2018, 33 human diseases could be prevented or substantially moderated by vaccination. Seventeen of these vaccines are routinely recommended for use in the United States. Routine vaccination helps prevent outbreaks of disease, protects individuals who for medical reasons cannot be vaccinated, and reduces health care costs. Vaccination of animals improves herd health, protects farmers' investments in their animals, and reduces the risk to humans of acquiring zoonotic diseases.

Pathogens that are easy to distribute widely and can kill or sicken many people quickly can be used as biological weapons. A substantial amount of research is directed toward development of vaccines against these pathogens. When a vaccine exists against a potential bioterrorism pathogen, the United States maintains stockpiles of this vaccine and other drugs for use during a bioterrorism attack or pandemic outbreak of disease.

The anti-vaccination movement attracts people from diverse backgrounds. Anti-vaccinationists believe that vaccines cause or have the potential to cause harm and that the decision to vaccinate should be an individual choice. They reject the CDC-recommended vaccination schedule.

About 28 percent of American children under age three have not received all the CDC-recommended inoculations for their age. Reasons for this deficit include medical conditions, lack access to health care, and deliberate choice by parents to not fully vaccinate. Vaccination requirements and ease of exemptions from vaccination in the United States are determined at the state level and vary considerably.

CHAPTER 2

Understanding the Immune System

Disease-causing pathogens and foreign irritants such as pollen are unavoidable. They are found by the millions in the air we breathe, the ground we walk on, the food we eat, and on the surfaces we touch. The body gives pathogens a good place to grow. It is warm and moist, contains plenty of nutrients, and has a circulatory system that makes it easy for pathogens to move around and settle in places where they can most successfully reproduce. Despite this, we rarely get sick. We stay healthy because our immune system effectively fights off most of these foreign invaders. This same ability to fight off foreign pathogens allows the body to develop immunity when inoculated with a vaccine.

The goal of vaccination is to develop long-term immunity against a disease caused by a specific organism without causing disease symptoms. To achieve this requires physical and chemical changes in the immune system and activation of a communication pathway that coordinates the response of individual cells and chemical reactions.

The immune system is the most widespread and complex system in the body. It differs from organ systems such as the digestive or nervous system because it is spread out among many different tissues and organs that are not physically connected. The immune system has multiple layers of defense against foreign invaders, and although it is not fully mature at birth, it still functions well, starting from day one.

FIRST LINES OF DEFENSE

The war against disease begins even before pathogens enter the body. Skin, the largest organ in the body, is the first line of defense. Its job is to keep pathogens out. When intact, skin forms a strong physical barrier between the outside world and the inside of the body, but even tiny breaks such as a paper cut can allow pathogens to enter and cause infection.

In addition to creating a physical barrier, skin has chemical defenses to discourage pathogens. Sebaceous skin glands secrete an oily, waxy substance that helps waterproof the skin and makes it harder for pathogens such as bacteria to enter. In addition, sweat from sweat glands makes the skin slightly acidic. The pH scale that measures acidity and alkalinity ranges from 1 to 14. A pH of 7 (the pH of pure water) is neutral. A pH of less than 7 is acidic. Sweat has a pH between 4 and 5.5. The acidity of the skin creates an environment that is hostile to many species of bacteria.

Some parts of the body exposed to the environment are lined with mucous membranes instead of skin. Mucous membrane is moist and lacks a waxy coating, making it easier for pathogens to penetrate. The sticky mucus in the mouth and the mucous membranes that line the airways can trap pathogens. Coughing and sneezing help to expel them. Mucus also contains antimicrobial proteins that kill or weaken some pathogens.

Tears and saliva wash away pathogens and contain chemicals that inhibit their growth. Vaginal secretions are slightly acidic to discourage microbial growth. Semen contains antimicrobial proteins and zinc that help kill some pathogens. Stomach acid, which has a pH between 1.5 and 3.0 (very acidic), kills many pathogens that are consumed in food. These mechanisms help prevent microbes from entering the bloodstream.

INTERNAL ORGANS AND TISSUES

The lymphatic system serves as the link among immune system tissues and organs. It consists of a series of branching channels or ducts separate from, but with connections to, the circulatory system. These channels move lymph, a colorless fluid that contains leukocytes (white blood cells), through the body. About 550 bean-shaped masses of tissue called lymph nodes are found along the lymph ducts in such places as the neck, under the arms, and in the groin. Lymph nodes filter and screen lymph for pathogens and abnormal cells.

Lymph nodes contain a high density of immune system cells that can destroy pathogens and abnormal body cells (e.g., cancer cells) that the nodes trap. When people talk about having swollen glands, they are really talking about enlarged lymph nodes that have been activated to fight disease. Lymph ducts connect with veins in the circulatory system so that lymph can mix with blood and immune system cells can reach all parts of the body. However, most immune system cells travel through the lymphatic system rather than the circulatory system.

All immune system cells begin life as stem cells in bone marrow. Bone marrow is a spongy material made up of blood vessels and connective tissue found mostly inside the ribs, sternum (breastbone), pelvis, and upper part of the long bones of the arms and legs. These bones contain a mix of two kinds of bone marrow. Red bone marrow contains stem cells that can become erythrocytes (red blood cells), leukocytes (white blood cells), or platelets (cells involved in blood clotting). Yellow bone marrow produces stem cells that become fat, bone, and cartilage.

Some leukocytes mature in the bone marrow. Others migrate to the thymus where they undergo maturation, and still others move into nonlymphoid tissues. The thymus is an immune system organ located above the heart and behind the breastbone. It produces proteins that help immune cells called T cells mature. The thymus is at its largest during puberty, weighing between 1 and 1.5 ounces (20–35 g). Starting in young adulthood, it begins to shrink and change into fatty tissue.

The spleen also has significant immune function. This brownish organ weighs about 6 ounces (170 g) and lies between the ninth and eleventh ribs on the left side of the abdomen. The spleen contains many blood vessels and lymph ducts. It acts as a filter, removing antibody-coated bacteria and damaged cells. The inner part of the spleen, known as the white pulp, contains a high density of antibody-producing leukocytes called B cells.

Tonsils, located in the back of the throat, and adenoids, located behind the nasal cavity, are lymphoid tissues that trap inhaled pathogens. Other clusters of lymphoid tissues are found in the appendix and in Peyer's patches, which are located in the lower portion of the small intestine. Sometimes, because of injury or infection, the spleen, tonsils, adenoids, or appendix must be removed. People can live without these organs, but their ability to fight infection is reduced.

DISTINGUISHING SELF FROM NONSELF

The immune system protects the body by attacking foreign antigens. To do this effectively, it must distinguish a person's healthy cells (self cells) from diseased or damaged self cells (sick self cells such as cancerous or virus-infected cells) and the millions of different pathogens (nonself cells or foreign antigens) that enter the body daily. The ability to attack only foreign material and leave healthy self cells unharmed is called immune tolerance.

Immune tolerance was first recognized by observing the results of early skin grafting operations. Doctors found that grafted donor skin usually was rejected by the recipient for no obvious reason such as infection. Eventually, researchers discovered that self cells with a nucleus (mature red blood cells are the main group that *do not* have nuclei) carry, or in the language of biology "express," a set of marker proteins on their surface called the major histocompatibility complex (MHC). In humans, MHC proteins are also called human leukocyte antigens (HLAs). No two humans express the exact same HLAs; even identical twins have minor differences in these proteins.

HLA molecules are antigens. They serve as a uniform that tells the immune system which cells are self cells. Cells without the proper self HLA proteins are identified as foreign or damaged and are targeted for destruction. Almost all early skin grafts were rejected because of a poor match between the donor's HLAs and the recipient's HLAs. As a result, the recipient's immune system identified the HLAs of the donated skin as foreign and destroyed it. Today, before skin grafts, bone marrow transplants, or organ transplants are performed, tests are done to match donor HLAs to recipient HLAs.

Pathogens also express identifying molecules on their surfaces. Since they are different from self cells' HLA markers, the immune system identifies pathogens as foreign and attacks them. The system for telling self from nonself is very effective, but it is not perfect. Some pathogens as well as sick self cells have evolved ways of escaping detection. Certain bacteria have a coating that protects them from being attacked and destroyed by immune system cells. Viruses enter healthy self cells where they are initially shielded from attack, and sick self cells may look enough like healthy cells to survive undetected. For vaccines to be effective, researchers must find ways to combat these evasion techniques.

Sometimes immune tolerance fails, and immune cells are inappropriately triggered to attack healthy self cells. When this happens, a person is said to have developed an autoimmune disorder. Common autoimmune disorders include multiple sclerosis, rheumatoid arthritis, systemic lupus erythematosus, and type 1 diabetes. Scientist do not yet understand what triggers the immune system to destroy healthy self cells, although clues suggest that some autoimmune disorders are associated with specific variations in genes that direct the production of cell surface proteins. People with autoimmune disorders or any other condition that weakens the immune system may not be able to safely receive some vaccines.

DIVISIONS OF THE IMMUNE SYSTEM

The immune system has two divisions that work together to fight infection: the innate immune system and the adaptive immune system. Both divisions are required to destroy pathogens. The relationship between the innate and the adaptive systems is complex, with some specialized immune cells acting as a communication bridge between the two divisions.

The Innate Immune System

The innate immune system is evolutionarily ancient. Elements of it are found in most living things. The system is called *innate* because it is present at birth and does not require any outside stimulation to develop. The innate immune system is quite similar in all healthy people.

Three characteristics define the innate immune system.

- Innate response is nonspecific. This means that the cells of the innate system recognize and respond in the same way to most pathogens, whether they are viruses, bacteria, or other foreign invaders. This occurs because many different of pathogens express on their surface an identical set of identifying antigens called pathogen-associated molecular patterns (PAMPs). PAMPs stimulate the same immune response from the innate system regardless of the species of pathogen.
- The innate system reacts quickly. The response begins as soon as the pathogen enters the body, and maximal response is reached within minutes to hours.
- The response of the innate system does not change no matter how often it encounters the same pathogen. Unlike the adaptive system, the innate system does not make memory cells and cannot develop immunological memory.

The Adaptive Immune System

The adaptive immune system, sometimes called the acquired immune system, is evolutionarily younger than the innate immune system. Complete adaptive immune response is found only in vertebrates with jaws, although some related elements of the system are found in other life forms. The system is called adaptive because unlike in the innate system, contact with pathogens causes long-term changes in the adaptive system response. While most people's innate system is nearly the same, their adaptive system varies based on the pathogens they have encountered.

Three characteristics distinguish the adaptive immune system from the innate immune system.

- The adaptive response is highly specific. Each cell (not each type of cell, but each single cell) in the adaptive immune system responds to only one antigen. That means an adaptive system cell attacks only one species or one strain of pathogen, while each innate cell can recognize and attack many different species of pathogens.
- The primary adaptive system response is slow. It takes about two weeks from first exposure to a pathogen to develop maximal response compared to the minutes to hours of the innate system response.
- When a pathogen has been destroyed, the adaptive system makes memory cells that remain in the body. This is the adaption part of the response. These memory cells can remember a pathogen and respond quickly when the same pathogen is encountered again. This remembered or secondary response takes about two to seven days. It is fast enough that the individual either does not become ill or has less severe symptoms the second time a pathogen invades. The rapid secondary response is what creates immunity to disease. Unlike the adaptive system, the innate system has no memory cells, and there is no change in its response no matter how often the same pathogen is encountered.

INNATE SYSTEM RESPONSE TO PATHOGEN PENETRATION

Cells of the innate immune system are the first to respond when a pathogen gets past the external defenses of skin and mucous membranes. As soon as the pathogen damages a body cell, the cell releases a chemical that acts as a call for help. The chemical sets off a cascading series of immune system actions and reactions. The chain of events is regulated by signaling molecules called cytokines and by the complement system. Cytokines are small molecules released by cells that control the behavior of other cells. The complement system (complement means to add to or supplement) consists of about 30 small proteins that circulate separately in the blood until a chemical message brings them together to form active molecules. The complement system controls actions and reactions of both innate and adaptive system cells.

The chemical distress signal released by damaged body cells calls leukocytes (white blood cells) to the injury site. As leukocytes begin to arrive, some cytokines signal additional immune cells to come to the area. Others increase blood flow to the wound so that more leukocytes can quickly reach the damaged area. Signaling molecules also make blood vessels near the injury site relax and become more permeable or leaky. This leakiness allows arriving immune system cells escape from the circulatory system and gather at the injured tissue.

As the response continues, other chemicals increase the temperature of the damaged tissue. Raising the temperature slows down pathogen growth. Soon the site of the injury becomes red, warm, and sore. This is a sign of local inflammation. More general signs of infection include fever, increased mucus production, runny nose, swollen joints, body aches, and local internal pain such as a sore throat or an ear ache. Although these signs make a person feel sick, they are positive indications that the immune system is working to control the pathogen.

Away from the site of infection, the bone marrow cranks up the production of leukocytes. After a few days, an increased number of leukocytes in the blood can be detected by a common laboratory test called a complete blood count or CBC. If the CBC shows an abnormally high white cell count, it is a positive indication the individual has an infection and that the immune system is trying to fight it.

CELLS OF THE INNATE IMMUNE SYSTEM

All immune system cells are leukocytes, but they have evolved into various specialized cells that perform different functions in defending the body. There are three classes of leukocytes in the innate system. Granulocytes are cells that contain packets or granules of destructive chemicals that they release to kill pathogens. Phagocytes are cells that change shape so that their cytoplasm flows around a pathogen and engulfs it. Once the pathogen is trapped inside the phagocyte, it is destroyed, a process called phagocytosis. Innate lymphocytes are leukocytes that have some characteristics of adaptive system cells but are considered part of the innate system.

Some cells classified as innate system cells such as macrophages and dendritic cells play crucial roles linking the innate and the adaptive system responses. In addition, many immune cells have other functions in the body such as mediating allergic reactions or preventing a woman's immune system from killing nonself fetal cells during pregnancy. The following discussion focuses only on the role these cells play in responding to a disease or a vaccine.

Granulocytes

Neutrophils are the most abundant leukocyte in the body and the first immune system cells to arrive at damaged tissue. Attracted by chemicals released from damaged cells, they migrate out of the bloodstream and into the damaged tissue within minutes. When they reach the site of tissue damage, neutrophils release signaling molecules to attract more cells to the area. They surround the pathogen and destroy it by releasing packets of chemicals with antimicrobial properties. This helps limit the spread of infection. Finally, these cells send out a spider web of filaments to trap pathogens and slow down their spread. Neutrophils die within one or two days but are quickly replaced because the body can make about 10 billion new neutrophils each day. Pus that accumulates at wound sites is made up mostly of dead neutrophils.

Eosinophils and basophils, two other types of granulocytes, also migrate to damaged tissues. Eosinophils release cytokines and enzymes that kill pathogens. These cells are most effective in controlling parasitic worms and are thought to play a role in fighting viral infections. Basophils contain large granules that release chemicals that increase blood flow and make blood vessels more permeable. They often gather at sites where external parasites such as ticks, lice, or fleas have broken the skin. Mast cells are similar to basophils and perform similar functions. They are more commonly associated with allergic reactions than with immune system response.

Phagocytes

Macrophages (literally "large eaters") are the clean-up crew of the immune system. Macrophages begin life in bone marrow as monocytes. They leave the bone marrow and travel through the bloodstream to many different tissues where they mature into macrophages. Macrophages clear the body of dead and dying cells. This is an ongoing function that does not require stimulation by immune system chemical signals. However, when a macrophage detects a chemical message from a damaged cell, it moves from its home tissue to the area of damage. Macrophages arrive at the infection site about 48 hours after neutrophils. They perform two jobs: clearing away dead and dying neutrophils and surrounding pathogens to destroy them through phagocytosis.

Once a macrophage has destroyed a pathogen, it takes a bit of the pathogen's antigenic protein and incorporates it into a molecule, which it then moves to its own cell surface. The process is called presenting the antigen. Now the macrophage looks to other immune cells like a foreign or nonself cell because it has the antigen of the pathogen on its surface. Antigen presentation is a link between the innate and the adaptive immune systems and an essential step in the production of antibodies and memory cells that create immunity.

Dendritic cells are also phagocytic antigen-presenting cells. They also serve as a crucial link between the innate and the adaptive immune systems. Dendritic cells were first identified in 1973 by Ralph Steinman (1943–2011), a Canadian immunologist. He named the cells for their tree-like branches; dendritic cells are not related to the similar-sounding dendrites found on nerve cells.

Immature dendritic cells are found in tissues that have contact with the outside environment such as skin and mucous membranes. These cells are hunters. They constantly search for invading pathogens, and when they find one, they phagocytize it and present the antigen. They then migrate to the thymus where the antigen activates a T cell that is part of the adaptive immune system.

Innate Lymphocytes

Natural killer (NK) cells straddle the line between the innate and the adaptive systems. They are classified as lymphocytes, as are T cells and B cells of the adaptive system, but are considered part of the innate system. NK cells mature in bone marrow and other lymphoid tissues such as the spleen, tonsil, thymus, and lymph nodes. Once mature, they enter the circulatory system.

NK cells do not directly kill pathogens. Instead, they recognize and kill damaged or altered self cells. These may be self cells that have been taken over by an invading virus or self cells that have become cancerous or otherwise been altered. Recent research also suggests that NK cells may have a memory function like the T and B memory cells (see The Adaptive Immune System) of the adaptive immune system. The cells of the innate immune system and their functions are summarized in Table 2.1.

Table 2.1 Cells of the Innate Immune System

Cell Name	Cell Type	Characteristics	Immune System Function
Neutrophil	Granulocyte	Most abundant leukocyte (60–70% of total leukocytes)	First responder to infection; especially responsive to bacterial infection and environmental toxins; also attacks fungi
Eosinophil	Granulocyte	Found in highest concentration in mucous membranes of respiratory, digestive, and urinary tracts	Attacks large parasites and bacteria

(Continued)

Table 2.1 (Continued)

Cell Name	Cell Type	Characteristics	Immune System Function
Basophil	Granulocyte	Least common leukocyte	Releases histamine to cause dilation of blood vessels and induce inflammatory response; attacks skin parasites
Mast cell	Granulocyte	Found in connective tissue, skin, and lining of digestive system	Releases histamine to cause dilation of blood vessels and induce inflammatory response; attacks internal parasites
Monocyte	Phagocyte	Immature macrophage	Develops into macrophage
Macrophage	Phagocyte	Largest leukocyte and antigen-presenting cell; links innate and adaptive immune systems	Engulfs pathogen, processes its protein, and presents it to T cells; removes dead and damaged neutrophils and pathogens
Dendritic cell	Phagocyte	Antigen-presenting cell; links innate and adaptive immune systems	Most efficient cell at engulfing a pathogen, processing it, and presenting it to T cells
Natural killer cell	Lymphocyte	Recognizes damaged self cells; part of both innate and adaptive immune systems	Removes virus-infected cells and tumor cells; may be retained as a type of memory cell

THE ADAPTIVE IMMUNE SYSTEM

When the innate immune system fails to contain a pathogen, the adaptive immune system kicks into high gear. The actions of two types of leukocytes, T lymphocytes (T cells) and B lymphocytes (B cells), are the mainstays of the adaptive system. The body contains between one and two trillion of these cells. If all the T and B cells were extracted from the body, their weight would be approximately equal to the weight of the brain. T and B cells have two main functions: (1) to rid the body of the invading pathogen, primarily by producing antibodies, and (2) to create long-lived memory cells that produce immunity to that specific pathogen.

Antigens and Antibodies

Antibodies, also called immunoglobulins (Igs), are tiny proteins produced by specialized B cells called plasma cells. While each cell in the innate system responds to many different pathogens, each cell in the adaptive system responds to only one unique antigen. As a result, in the adaptive system, antigens and antibodies work like a lock and key. Every antibody has a binding site that will fit only with a matching antigen. This means that every antibody produced by the adaptive system can bind to and inactivate the antigen of only one species or subspecies of pathogen. There are five classes of antibodies (IgA, IgD, IgE, IgG, IgM), each with a different immune function.

Creating Antibody Diversity

The world is full of millions of pathogens. Scientists estimate that adaptive system cells can recognize up to 100 million different antigens and make antibodies against all of them. Researchers have even created artificial antigens not found in nature and shown that they stimulate the immune system to make antibodies against them.

The human genome contains only about 20,000 genes. Given what scientists know about DNA recombination and genetic diversity, one would predict that it would take many more genes to code for the number of unique T cells and B cells needed to recognize millions of different antigens. How can such a small genome create so much diversity? The answer lies in the structure of the antibody and a special process of shuffling DNA called somatic diversification or VDJ (variable diversity joining) recombination.

VDJ recombination occurs early in the maturation process of T cells and B cells and nowhere else in the body. In T cells, VDJ is responsible for the rearrangement of the genetic material that creates a unique receptor on the surface of each T cell. In B cells, VDJ is responsible for the shuffling of genetic material to produce antibodies, each capable of interacting with only one type of antigen.

Antibodies are shaped like a Y. The stem, or vertical part of the Y, has only five different forms. All antibodies in the same class (IgA, IgD, IgE, IgG, IgM) have the same stem. The V-shaped arms of the Y are made up of two parallel chains of proteins linked by sulfur bonds (S–S). VDJ recombination occurs in the genes that control the proteins found in the arms. The end of the arms is where antibody–antigen binding occurs. See Figure 2.1.

In VDJ recombination, only three gene segments are involved. Each segment contains multiple bits of genetic material—about 40 V bits, 30 D bits, and 6 J bits. Through the action of enzymes, one bit from each segment is randomly snipped out and combined in each developing T or B cell to produce genetic material that will direct the production of a unique T cell receptor or B cell antibody. The genetic material not selected plays no role

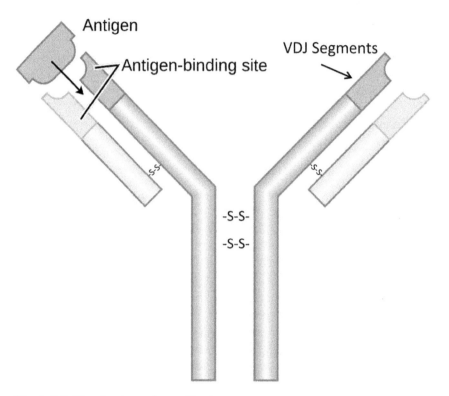

Figure 2.1 The structure of an antibody

(Adapted from National Institutes of Health. National Human Genome Research Institute. "Talking Glossary of Genetic Terms." Online at https://www.genome.gov/glossary/).

in this process and is snipped away by other enzymes. All the possible VDJ combinations for both arms plus five different stems add up to more than 400 million possible combinations. This is more than enough variety to recognize every antigen an individual is exposed to during a lifetime.

The V, D, and J gene segments are also areas of hypermutation. This means that the sequence of base pairs that make up the DNA for these regions undergoes spontaneous change much more often than occurs in other parts of the gene. Recombination and hypermutation allow immune system cells to adapt to the antigens of newly evolving pathogens whose surface proteins are unlike any they have encountered before.

The Role of T Cells

T cells arise from stem cells in bone marrow and while still immature migrate to the thymus. In the thymus, they undergo VDJ recombination.

This results in each T cell having a unique surface receptor. The T cell receptor is like a lock in which only one specific antigen will work as a key.

When a dendritic cell migrates to the thymus, it presents its antigen to the T cells gathered there. If the dendritic cell meets a T cell whose receptor matches the dendritic cell's antigen, the cells bind, and the T cell becomes a functional immune system cell.

Through random VDJ recombination, some T cells develop receptors that match the proteins (HLAs) on the surface of healthy self cells. If these T cells were to circulate in the body, they would destroy normal, healthy cells. To prevent the body from destroying its own cells, all T cells with receptors matching self cell surface proteins die before they can leave the thymus. The process that causes them to die is not well understood.

Cytotoxic T Leukocytes

Based on their surface protein markers, there are two major subtypes of T cells and several minor subtypes, all with different immune functions. One major T cell subtype has the CD8 protein on its surface. In the thymus, when a dendritic cell activates a CD8+ T cell (the + indicates the presence of the protein), the cell undergoes clonal expansion. During clonal expansion, the cell divides repeatedly to create a huge number of identical CD8+ daughter cells. These cells become cytotoxic T leukocytes (CTLs), also referred to as killer T cells. CTLs leave the thymus and enter the bloodstream. When they encounter a foreign cell with an antigen that matches their receptor, they bind to that cell and destroy it.

Helper T Cells

T cells with the CD4 surface protein are also activated by dendritic cells. These T cells undergo clonal expansion, creating many CD4+ daughter cells, but the CD4+ cells become T helper (TH) cells. TH cells leave the thymus and migrate to the site of infection. Unlike CTLs, TH cells cannot directly kill pathogens. Instead, they secrete chemicals that communicate instructions to other immune system cells. Some of these chemicals help B cells differentiate into antibody-secreting plasma cells. Others help CTLs mature into active killers. A select group of TH cells matures into memory T cells.

Memory T Cells

Besides the specificity of the adaptive immune system, its other special characteristic is its ability to create a data bank of cells that remember specific antigens and respond quickly if the antigen is encountered later in life. To develop this data bank, the body creates memory cells. Some T cells, instead of being activated as functional CTLs or THs, become long-lived memory T cells. Scientists are still unraveling the exact process by which memory cells are formed. They have identified at least three different types of memory T cells that are distinguished by their surface proteins and the chemicals they secrete. Understanding how memory cells are made and activated is important to vaccine research because these cells can remain in the body for years and are the cornerstone for conferring immunity to disease.

Regulatory T Cells

Once a pathogen has been cleared from the body, the immune response needs to wind down. Regulatory T cells (Tregs), also called suppressor T cells, play a role in stopping the activities of other immune cells. About 10 percent of CD4+ helper cells become Tregs. Although their role is not well understood, Tregs appear to strip antigen-presenting cells of their antigen, thus stopping the adaptive immune response. They also may kill active CTLs by binding with them and releasing destructive chemicals. Table 2.2 summarizes the cells of the adaptive immune system.

Table 2.2 Cells of the Adaptive Immune System

Cell Name	Cell Type	Cell Function
Cytotoxic T cell (CD8+ cell)	T lymphocyte	Directly kills virus- or bacteria-infected cells and abnormal cells through the release of toxins
Helper T cell (CD4+ cell)	T lymphocyte	Releases cytokines that direct the action of other immune cells and activate antibody formation by B cells
Regulatory T cell	T lymphocyte	Releases chemicals that wind down the immune response once a pathogen has been controlled and prevents immune response against self cells
Memory T cell	T lymphocyte	T cell that remains in the body after a pathogen has been eliminated until activated by a second encounter with the pathogen
Plasma cell	B lymphocyte	Secretes antibodies after stimulation by helper T cell
Memory B cell	B lymphocyte	B cell that remains in the body after a pathogen has been eliminated until activated by a second encounter with the pathogen

The Role of B Cells

B cells, like T cells, arise from stem cells in the bone marrow. Unlike T cells, B cells do not migrate but undergo VDJ recombination and mature in bone marrow. In contrast to T cells, B cells recognize foreign antigens directly when they encounter them in blood and lymph; they do not need to have the antigen engulfed, processed, and presented to them to be activated.

Once a B cell receptor binds to a matching antigen, the B cell is activated and begins to divide. Most of the resulting identical daughter B cells become plasma cells. Plasma cells secrete antibody molecules directly into the blood and lymph at the astounding rate of 2,000 per second for three to five days. These antibodies are identical, and they are specific to the antigen that activated the mother B cell.

With help from the complement system, antibodies can hook together multiple pathogens making them bigger targets and thus easier for phagocytes to destroy. In conjunction with chemical signals from the complement system, antibodies can also make pathogens more susceptible to destruction by macrophages, or they can bind directly to the pathogen so that it can no longer attach to and damage healthy body cells. Some bacteria release toxins that cause illnesses such as diphtheria and tetanus. These toxins act as antigens. B cells can make antibodies against them and block the site of toxin production.

Memory B Cells

Not all B cells become antibody-producing plasma cells. Under the direction of chemicals released by TH cells, some B cells become memory B cells. Like memory T cells, the formation of memory B cells is not completely understood. Memory B cells play a critical role in adaptive immunity. They remain in the body for a long time and respond promptly by producing a swarm of antibodies when challenged by a pathogen they have already met. The capacity to recognize a repeat pathogen and respond to it rapidly keeps that individual from becoming sick a second time from the same pathogen.

TYPES OF IMMUNITY

So far, we have discussed how the body makes memory cells to develop immunity to a disease. This type of self-made long-term immunity is called active immunity. Another type of immunity called passive immunity depends on acquiring antibodies from an outside source. Unlike active immunity, passive immunity is always temporary. Herd immunity is a third type of immunity that involves an entire community. Although vaccines are concerned with developing active immunity, other types of immunity sometimes figure into the calculation vaccine-skeptic parents make in deciding whether or when to vaccinate their children.

Active Immunity

Active immunity results from the formation immunological memory through the creation of memory T cells and memory B cells. Natural active immunity develops when an individual becomes infected with a pathogen, gets sick, and then recovers. In artificial active immunity, the antigens in a vaccine substitute for infection with a pathogen. The antigens in the vaccine are strong enough to create memory cells but weakened enough not to cause illness. The immune system's response to antigens in a vaccine may not be as strong or long lasting as it is toward a naturally acquired pathogen; consequently, multiple doses of vaccine may be needed to create and maintain immunity.

Passive Immunity

Passive immunity involves "borrowing" antibodies. When a baby is born, it has an immature immune system, no prior exposure to external pathogens, and no memory cells. Instead, an infant is partially protected by antibodies acquired from its mother during fetal development. This type of immunity is designated naturally acquired passive immunity because it happens without any medical intervention and it is short term; no memory cells are made.

Only two of the five classes of antibodies (IgA and IgG) participate in the creation of naturally acquired passive immunity. Beginning around the third month of pregnancy, maternal IgG antibodies cross the placenta and enter the fetus. IgG is the only class of antibodies transferred to the fetus during development, but this class makes up about 80 percent of all antibodies. When the baby is born, it has the same IgG antibodies as its mother. If, for example, the mother is immune to measles, the baby will have temporary immunity to measles. However, if the mother has not had natural measles or been vaccinated against the disease, the baby will have no protection.

Another class of antibodies, IgA, is passed from mother to child in breast milk. IgA antibodies provide the newborn with passive immunity mainly to pathogens found in the digestive system. The baby will have protection only against diseases that the mother has made memory cells against and only if the infant is breast fed. Because of natural passive immunity, babies born to fully vaccinated mothers have better protection against disease early in life than babies of incompletely vaccinated mothers.

Passive immunity is always temporary because no memory T or B cells are made and no immunological memory is created. In infants, transferred passive immunity lasts from a few days to several months. The period during which the maternal antibodies remain effective and the rate at which the newborn's immune system matures are taken into account when the Centers for Disease Control and Prevention (CDC) develops its recommended childhood vaccination schedule.

Artificial passive immunity can also be created through medical intervention. Like natural passive immunity, the benefit is short term and no memory cells are made. Artificially acquired passive immunity can be created by injecting blood plasma or serum (the clear part of the blood that contains antibodies) from a person or an animal that has developed antibodies to the disease being treated. For example, during the Ebola virus outbreak in 2014, antibodies from patients who had recovered from Ebola infection were given to actively infected patients in the hope of improving their chance of survival.

Artificial passive immunity can also be induced by the injection of monoclonal antibodies. Monoclonal antibodies are identical, laboratory-produced antibodies derived from a single cell that has been cloned to produce millions of genetically identical daughter cells. Monoclonal antibodies are used most often to treat cancers and autoimmune diseases. They are not used to treat vaccine-preventable diseases.

Herd Immunity

Herd immunity, sometimes called community immunity, is the situation that arises when many people or animals within a specific area have been vaccinated against a disease. With many disease-resistant individuals in a community, the chain of pathogen transmission is broken so that the entire community is protected from epidemic illness. The more infectious the disease, the higher the percentage of individuals who need to be disease-resistant to create herd immunity. Epidemiologists—scientists who study disease transmission—rate how transmissible a disease is by estimating the average number of people a single sick person will infect. From that, they determine what percentage of the population must be disease-resistant to create herd immunity.

Measles and pertussis (whooping cough) are the most transmissible of the vaccine-preventable diseases. A single person infected with either disease will infect between 12 and 18 other people. This translates into needing 92–94 percent of the population to be vaccinated to stop the spread of either disease. Tetanus is the only vaccine-preventable disease where herd immunity does not apply. It is caused by the toxins of a bacterium found in soil and manure. It is never transmitted from person to person.

Some people who choose not to vaccinate do so with the belief that herd immunity will protect them or their children from getting sick. This may be true if enough people in their community are vaccinated. Nevertheless, unvaccinated individuals who live in or move to an area where the vaccination rates are low or who travel abroad to areas where a disease is active will be vulnerable to becoming ill and then spreading disease to others.

MEASURING IMMUNE RESPONSE

How can researchers know if a vaccine works without waiting for a disease outbreak to monitor who gets sick and who does not? An antibody titer test performed a few weeks after a vaccine has been administered will give the answer. Antibody titer tests measure the amount of a specified antibody in blood serum. The quantity of antibodies present in the blood indicates the strength of the immune response. A strong response is highly correlated to the production of memory cells and the development of immunity.

An antibody titer is calculated by a series of dilutions. First, one part blood serum is added to two parts diluting solution and the antibodies are measured. Next, one part serum is added to four parts diluting serum, then eight parts diluting solution, and so on until it is no longer possible to detect a measurable number of antibodies in the solution. The titer value is the last degree of dilution at which measurable antibodies were present. A strong immune response to a vaccine results in a high titer value, while a poor response results in a low number.

Because the effectiveness of some vaccines decreases over time, antibody titer tests can also be used to determine how long immunity lasts. This is done by measuring the quantity of antibodies present at set time intervals, for example, every six months or every year. When the titer falls below a certain number, a booster shot is needed to maintain immunity. Weakening of immunity over time is considered when developing the CDC-recommended vaccination schedule.

Antibody titer tests can also show whether an unvaccinated person has already acquired natural active immunity by having a disease and recovering. In this case, the level of antibodies in the blood will be high, and vaccination is unnecessary. Some parents who choose to have their children to skip certain inoculations (often measles and chickenpox) request an anti-body titer test for these diseases when their children reach about age 12. The test will show if the child has acquired natural immunity to the disease. If not, parents may then choose to vaccinate because these diseases cause more serious symptoms and complications in teens and adults than they do in younger children.

LIMITATIONS OF VACCINES

No vaccines are 100 percent effective in every individual, nor are they completely without health risks, although serious health complications are extremely rare. Almost everyone who is inoculated makes some antibodies to a vaccine, but some people do not make enough to prevent the disease. Consequently, a few people still get sick from a disease they have been vaccinated against. People can also fall ill after vaccination if they are already infected with the disease the vaccine is intended to prevent but have not yet developed symptoms at the time of vaccination. This happens most often with pathogens that have a long incubation period. With measles, for example, after infection, it takes 7–21 days for a rash to appear. This leads some already-infected people to believe that the vaccine has caused the disease.

Overall, routine childhood vaccinations are about 90 percent effective. This means nine out of ten fully vaccinated children will not get a vaccine-preventable disease. Failure to receive all the required doses is a major cause of reduced immunity. For some diseases (e.g., diphtheria, tetanus), the effectiveness of the vaccine diminishes over time. To maintain immunity, revaccination or booster shots are needed many years after initial immunization. Adult vaccinations are less effective than childhood vaccinations, because as people age, their immune system responds less strongly to vaccines. Adults often make enough antibodies to lessen disease symptoms but not to completely prevent illness.

The influenza vaccine is the least-effective vaccine. Effectiveness generally ranges from 40 percent to 60 percent. The 2016–2017 vaccine had an effective rate of 42 percent, and initial data suggested the 2017–2018 rate would be around 32 percent. The influenza virus mutates rapidly, creating different strains of the pathogen. Each year, the composition of the vaccine changes to contain antigens of three or four different flu strains based on data from a worldwide influenza-tracking system. Consequently, people need to be vaccinated against influenza each year. The decision about which strains to include must be made well in advance of flu season. When the match between influenza strains circulating in a community is good, the vaccine is highly effective. When the match is poor, people become sick from strains not included in the vaccine.

From the discussion in this chapter, it is clear that the immune system is a complex defense system designed to defeat pathogens. It begins functioning at birth to destroy disease-causing pathogens. A characteristic of all immune system cells is that they can distinguish self cells from nonself cells. Human cells carry identifying marker proteins called HLAs on their surface that are different from the marker proteins (antigens) on the surface of nonself cells. In a healthy person, immune cells attack only nonself cells or sick and damaged self cells. Sometimes, this recognition system breaks down and the immune system attacks self cells. When this occurs, the individual develops an autoimmune disease.

Skin and mucus membranes provide physical and chemical barriers to pathogens. Internal organs of the immune system include the thymus, spleen, tonsils, adenoids, appendix, and Peyer's patches.

The immune system has two divisions that work together to kill pathogens. When pathogens get past external barriers, the innate immune system responds immediately. The innate system consists of three varieties of cells: granulocytes, phagocytes, and innate lymphocytes. These cells respond rapidly when pathogens penetrate the body. Their response is the same no matter how often they encounter the same pathogen. The sequence of events needed for these cells to destroy a pathogen is directed by signaling chemicals and the complement system.

Macrophages and dendritic cells of the innate system act as a bridge between the innate and the adaptive immune systems. The adaptive system consists of T cells and B cells, of which there are various subtypes with different functions. Adaptive system response is slow (days) and highly specific. Some T cells kill pathogens, while others secrete chemicals that direct the actions of other cells. B cells produce antibodies that can bind only to the antigen of a specific pathogen. Through a special shuffling of genetic material called VDJ recombination that happens only in B and T cells, these cells can recognize millions of different antigens.

Both T cells and B cells form memory cells that remain in the body long after a pathogen has been defeated. Memory cells are the basis for immunological memory that creates immunity. When a pathogen is re-encountered later in life, memory cells stimulate the immune system to respond quickly so that the individual does not become sick or has a less severe illness.

There are multiple types of immunity. Active immunity is developed by exposure to a pathogen or a vaccine that contains a pathogen's antigens, resulting in the creation of memory cells. Active immunity is long lasting.

Passive immunity occurs when antibodies are passed from one person to another as from mother to fetus or through medical intervention. Passive immunity is temporary. Herd immunity occurs when so many individuals have immunity to a disease (usually through vaccination) that transmission of the pathogen is interrupted and unvaccinated individuals may be protected from becoming sick.

Childhood vaccines are, on average, 90 percent effective if given in accordance with the CDC-recommended vaccination schedule. Response to a vaccination can be determined using antibody titer tests that measure the amount of antibodies in the blood.

CHAPTER 3

Making Vaccines

Making a vaccine is difficult. It takes, on average, 10–15 years and many millions of dollars to bring a new vaccine to market. In the United States, production of vaccines is regulated under federal law. Regulations have changed over time to keep up with new technology and an increased public demand for assurances of safety. More changes are likely as the ability to use genetic engineering to produce vaccines advances. Federal regulations affecting vaccines are discussed in Chapter 4.

DEVELOPING A VACCINE

The perfect vaccine would stimulate lifelong immunity with a single dose and no undesirable side effects in 100 percent of people vaccinated. There are no ideal vaccines. Vaccine developers must balance a variety of medical and nonmedical factors to get as close to the ideal vaccine as possible. As a result, vaccines against the same diseases are manufactured using different techniques to create products with multiple routes of administration that require varying dosage schedules. The following are some of the medical and biological issues that must be considered during vaccine development.

- The type of pathogen: Vaccines against bacterial diseases are harder to make than vaccines against viral diseases, and as of 2018, no successful vaccine has been licensed against a parasitic disease such as malaria or a fungal disease.
- The level of adverse effects the vaccine causes: Adverse effects are undesirable reactions that are proven to be caused by the vaccine.

Most are mild, such as soreness and redness at the injection site. No vaccine will be completely free of all adverse effects in every person because of human genetic variability, but for a vaccine to be successful, serious adverse effects must be on the order of one or two per million doses.

- The number and timing of doses needed to achieve and maintain immunity: The biology of some pathogens makes it more difficult to stimulate an adequate immune response. It may take multiple doses of vaccine and booster shots to achieve and maintain immunity against these pathogens.
- The speed at which a pathogen mutates: HIV and the influenza virus mutate frequently, while the measles virus barely changes. A vaccine against a virus that mutates often may be effective today and close to useless within a few years.
- The population to be vaccinated: Some vaccines do not stimulate the immune system of very young children enough to create immunity. The immune system of older individuals responds less strongly to vaccines than the immune system of younger people. Some people have health conditions or are taking medications that change the effectiveness of the vaccine, and if a pregnant woman is vaccinated, the effect of the vaccine on the fetus must be considered.

In addition to medical factors related to vaccine development, the following nonmedical issues must be considered when producing a vaccine on a commercial scale.

- Ease of scaling up production to a commercial level: It may be relatively easy to make enough vaccine in the laboratory for a few dozen people during early clinical trials, but it is more difficult to produce millions of doses needed to vaccinate a large segment of the population.
- Expected lifetime: A vaccine can be stored only for a limited time before it loses potency, becomes unstable, and must be discarded.
- Conditions under which the vaccine must be kept: Exposure to light, heat, and temperature fluctuations must be controlled and monitored. Many vaccines must remain continuously refrigerated within a very limited temperature range from the time of manufacture through transport, storage, and use. The Ebola vaccine used to combat an outbreak in the Democratic Republic of the Congo in 2018 had to be kept at a temperature between –60°C and –80°C (–76°F and –112°F) to maintain its effectiveness. Some vaccines lose potency

when exposed to normal room temperature for as little as 30 minutes. A continuous cold chain can be difficult to maintain if the vaccine is used in areas where the electrical supply is inconsistent or when transportation delays are severe, such as during a natural disaster. The World Health Organization (WHO) estimates the need to maintain the cold chain increases the cost of immunization programs by 14 percent, and that one-quarter to one-half of all vaccines the WHO distributes must be destroyed because of breaks in the cold chain.

• Ease and cost of transport and storage: Single-dose syringes reduce the risk of contamination and can be preservative-free, but they add significantly to the cost of distribution and storage. The WHO estimates that five times more cold storage space is needed for single-dose syringes than for 10- and 20-dose vials, but multiuse vials require the addition of preservatives.

• Ease of administration: Most vaccines are given by injection, which requires trained health care workers, sterile needles, and appropriate needle disposal. Vaccines that can be given orally or as a nasal spray or perhaps in the future as a skin patch do not have these limitations.

Balancing competing biological and production factors has resulted in the development of multiple vaccines against the same disease to meet the needs of different populations. For example, inactivated polio vaccine (IPV) is used in the United States. IPV is given by injection, contains no live *poliovirus,* and cannot cause polio. Oral polio vaccine (OPV), which contains live attenuated (weakened) *poliovirus,* is used in the developing world. Because OPV contains live virus, it can cause polio once in about every 2.7 million doses. However, OPV is approved by the WHO because the advantages of an easy-to-administer oral vaccine outweigh the minimal risk of the live attenuated virus causing polio.

LIVE ATTENUATED VACCINES

Live attenuated vaccines contain living viruses or bacteria that have been weakened to the point where they do not cause the disease but still stimulate the immune system to create antibodies and memory cells. The concept of putting a weakened variant of a virus that causes serious disease to a healthy person to protect that person from that same disease can be difficult to accept. Nevertheless, this approach to creating immunity works because the weakened virus retains its distinctive antigenic surface molecules. The immune system recognizes the surface molecules as nonself and makes antibodies and memory cells against them. At the same time, the virus has been made so weak that it cannot reproduce efficiently enough to cause illness.

Attenuating a pathogen is done by growing it in a hostile environment. Viruses cannot reproduce on their own. To reproduce, they must enter a host cell and take over the cell's metabolic machinery to produce new virus particles (virons). This is the equivalent of an army invading a car manufacturing plant, rearranging all the machinery, and starting to produce tanks.

Viruses that infect humans are highly adapted to taking over human cells. However, if the virus is grown in nonhuman cells (often fertilized chicken eggs), at first it will not be very successful in invading these new cells. Many virons will die, but because of genetic variability, some will have mutations that allow them to invade the new cell type and reproduce vigorously.

As generations of virons reproduce in the nonhuman cells, natural selection makes them progressively better adapted to infecting the new cell type and less well adapted to infecting human cells. Eventually when enough generations have passed, the virus infecting the nonhuman cells will have changed so much that it is too weak to cause disease in humans. However, some of the mutated virons will retain their original surface proteins. Those virons can still stimulate the human immune system to make antibodies and memory cells against the disease they originally caused, but they do this without making people sick. This is the basis for immunity created by live attenuated vaccines. One or two doses of a live attenuated vaccine provide strong long-lasting immunity. Viral diseases prevented by live attenuated vaccines include adenovirus, chickenpox, measles, mumps, rotavirus, rubella shingles, and yellow fever.

Bacteria are much harder to attenuate than viruses. How much harder? Consider the work of Léon Charles Albert Calmette (1863–1933), a French navy doctor, and Camille Guérin (1872–1961), a veterinarian, who worked together in the early 1900s to create a live attenuated tuberculosis (TB) vaccine. They began with the bacterium *Mycobacterium bovis,* which causes TB in cows and is closely related to *M. tuberculosis,* the bacterium that causes human TB.

Bacteria can reproduce on their own; they do not need to enter a host cell. To attenuate them, they are grown in cultures that provide an unfavorable environment in which natural selection can work. First Calmette and Guérin tried growing the bacterium in a mixture of glycerin and potato, but the bacteria clumped too much to be useful. To counteract this, they added bile from the gallbladders of oxen to the culture. Ox bile successfully prevented clumping and weakened the bacterium, which was an advantage in achieving attenuation.

Beginning in 1908, and every three weeks for the next 13 years, Calmette and Guérin transferred the bacteria to a new batch of culture to progressively weaken it. By 1913, they had a vaccine ready to test a vaccine on cattle, but World War I (1914–1918) erupted and threatened end to their research. German troops occupied France, and Calmette and Guérin were no longer able to obtain enough ox bile to keep their culture alive. It looked as if 13 years of work would become a casualty of war. Fortunately, their culture was saved when German veterinary surgeons agreed to collect bile for them from slaughterhouses.

By the end of the war, after years of work and 230 culture transfers, Calmette and Guérin had created a live attenuated bacterial vaccine that protected guinea pigs, rabbits, cattle, and horses against TB. They named their vaccine Bacille Calmette-Guérin or BCG. The first test of BCG in humans occurred in 1921. It was a success, and almost 100 years later, BCG vaccine is still used in many countries where TB is common. The only other live attenuated bacterial vaccines in use today are plague vaccine and one form of typhoid vaccine.

INACTIVATED OR KILLED VACCINES

Inactivated or killed vaccines are created by making the pathogen inactive or dead so that it is unable to reproduce. Inactivated refers to viral pathogens. Viruses cannot reproduce on their own and are not considered living organisms, so they cannot be killed. Killed refers to bacterial pathogens because bacteria are living organisms. Inactivation/killing is done by exposing the pathogen to heat or chemicals, often a dilute solution of formaldehyde (formalin). With both inactivated and killed vaccines, the pathogen cannot reproduce inside the body, cannot mutate, and cannot cause disease.

Inactivated/killed pathogens keep their distinctive surface antigens and still stimulate the immune system to make antibodies and memory cells. The immune response is weaker than with a vaccine made from live attenuated pathogens. Multiple doses and booster shots of an inactivated/killed vaccine are needed to achieve and maintain immunity. Inactivated/killed vaccines include hepatitis A, inactivated influenza vaccine (IIV), Japanese encephalitis (although a live attenuated vaccine is used in China), whole cell pertussis (not the form used in the United States), IPV, and rabies.

Inactivated/killed vaccines have certain advantages. They are safer than live attenuated vaccines because then can never mutate or cause disease. They may not need to be kept under strict cold chain conditions. This reduces transport and storage costs and makes them more accessible to people in developing countries. To assure safety, every batch of inacti-vated/killed vaccine must be tested to verify that no active/living patho-gens have survived. This was not always the law, and the result was a vaccine tragedy known as the Cutter incident.

The Cutter Incident

In the summer of 1952, an epidemic of polio swept across the United States. The disease was a parent's nightmare. In severe cases, *poliovirus* destroys the gray matter of the spinal cord, which contains nerve cells that relay signals essential for muscle coordination. A child could go to bed feeling mildly ill and wake up paralyzed. By the time the 1952 epidemic was over, 21,269 people had been left with permanent paralysis and 3,145 others were dead. The pressure was on to find a vaccine to prevent future epidemics.

The National Foundation for Infantile Paralysis (NFIP, now called the March of Dimes) was in charge organizing research for a polio vaccine. To help fund the project, the NFIP encouraged ordinary citizens to send one dime to the White House in honor of the birthday of President Franklin D. Roosevelt (1882–1945), the best-known adult victim of par-alytic polio. Americans were so eager to have a polio vaccine that, by the time the campaign ended, they had sent the White House $250,000 in dimes, the equivalent of about $2.3 million in 2018 dollars.

Jonas Salk (1914–1995) and his research team worked diligently to develop an IPV. His competitor, Albert Sabin (1906–1993), led a team developing a live attenuated vaccine (now called oral polio vaccine, OPV). Although Sabin was eventually successful, Salk's vaccine was perfected first. Salk considered his vaccine a gift to the American people and refused to personally profit from it. He became a national hero, and Sabin became an angry, bitter man who resented Salk for the rest of his life.

Salk's team made IPV by growing *poliovirus* in monkey kidney cells, inactivating it with formalin, and then filtering and purifying the inactive virus. By 1953, Salk was so confident his vaccine was safe and effective that he vaccinated himself, his wife, and his three children. No one in the family showed any negative effects from the vaccine.

The following year, the Salk polio vaccine was ready for a large field trial. Parents eagerly volunteered their children as participants. Eventu-ally 440,000 people were vaccinated, and the results compared with those of an equally large unvaccinated control group. On April 12, 1955, the vaccine field test was declared a success. Within hours, the Laboratory of Biologics Control, a federal agency within the National Institutes of Health, signed off on a license for the vaccine. The news caused a sensation. Church bells rang in celebration, and the story of Salk's success headlined practically every newspaper in America.

The NFIP had anticipated that there would be a stampede of parents wanting to get the new vaccine for their children as soon as it was licensed. To meet the expected demand, the NFIP had unconditionally contracted with five laboratories to make 27 million doses of polio vaccine at a cost of $9 million ($82 million in 2018 dollars) while the field trial was under way. If the vaccine had failed the trial, the NFIP would pay the laboratories for the vaccine and destroy it. But the vaccine was a success, and all five laboratories began shipping their stockpiled vaccine immediately.

Cutter Laboratory, in Berkeley, California, was one of the laboratories chosen to make the vaccine. Cutter had trouble inactivating the *poliovirus* early in production. When it tested the finished vaccine, it found that some batches still contained live virus. Cutter destroyed these batches, but it never told the NFIP or any government agency connected with the vaccine project about its production problems.

At the time, what Cutter did was legal. No law required manufacturers to report test results on batches of vaccine not released to the public. However, some batches of Cutter vaccine containing live virus slipped undetected through the testing process. As soon as the polio vaccine was licensed, Cutter's vaccine was shipped to doctors across the country and used to vaccinate about 400,000 children.

Twelve days after Salk's polio vaccine had been declared a success, a vaccinated child in Idaho contracted polio and died. Soon there were reports of children in other parts of the country developing polio after vaccination. The public panicked when the news got out that the polio vaccine was causing polio. The government stopped the vaccination program less than one month after it had begun, but not before 94 children contracted polio from Cutter vaccine. No children were infected by vaccine made by the other four laboratories. The children infected by Cutter vaccine spread the disease to other people. Of the 260 people whose polio could be traced to Cutter vaccine, 192 had permanent paralysis and 11 died.

Once Cutter Laboratory was pinpointed as the source of the problem, the vaccination program was restarted without Cutter vaccine. Understandably, parents were left confused about the risks of a vaccine they had so enthusiastically welcomed and questioned whether they should risk having their children vaccinated. It did not help that Cutter never accepted blame for the polio their vaccine caused. The company insisted that it had followed the information and procedures it was given and claimed that it had become the scapegoat for failures in the program. No one at Cutter lost his or her job after this disaster. Conversely, everyone in the government involved in testing and licensing of the polio vaccine, from laboratory scientists all the way up to the Secretary of the Department of Health, Education, and Welfare, was fired.

After the Cutter incident, the government tightened rules regulating vaccine manufacture. Record keeping became stricter. Today companies must report test results of every batch, even those not released to the public. Tightening the rules regulating vaccine production has prevented another Cutter-like incident from occurring. Nevertheless, the Cutter experience demonstrates the need for rigorous production oversight and illustrates the disastrous consequences of failing to completely inactivate a virus used in an inactivated vaccine.

Toxoid Vaccines

In some cases, illness is caused not by a pathogen but by the poisonous waste product (toxin) that it produces. This is true of the vaccine-preventable diseases diphtheria and tetanus. *Corynebacterium diphtheriae,* the bacterium that causes diphtheria, is breathed in and sticks to the cells lining the airways. The airway cells are damaged by toxins released by the bacteria. Soon a membrane forms made of dead cells and fibrin, a protein that helps blood clot. The membrane can be large enough to cut off air supply to the lungs. Before there was an effective diphtheria vaccine, 20 percent children younger than five years and up to 10 percent of older people who contracted the disease died.

The *Clostridium tetani* bacterium that causes tetanus (also called lockjaw) releases a toxin that makes muscles spasm painfully and become paralyzed. Up to three-quarters of people who develop tetanus cannot open their jaw, and about 10 percent die when muscles needed to breathe are paralyzed. Unlike many vaccine-preventable diseases, having tetanus and recovering does not provide permanent immunity. The only way to become immune is through vaccination and lifelong regular booster shots, usually at 10-year intervals.

Toxoid vaccines are made by growing huge numbers of the pathogen in the laboratory. The pathogen secretes toxin into the growth medium. The growth medium is then filtered and the toxin purified. Next, it is neutralized by exposure to formalin or heat. The neutralized toxin does not cause disease but still stimulates the immune system to make memory cells. Diphtheria and tetanus are the only toxoid vaccines given to humans, but a toxoid vaccine against rattlesnake poison is available for dogs.

Subunit Vaccines

Subunit vaccines get their name because they contain only antigenic proteins of a pathogen, not the whole organism. Because the organism is not present, subunit vaccines cannot cause disease. Eliminating the whole organism helps reduce undesirable side effects and increases the stability of the vaccine. Most subunit vaccines contain between 1 and 20 antigenic proteins. The main drawback to subunit vaccines is that they may not stimulate a strong enough immune system response to create immunological memory. Subunit vaccines include anthrax, hepatitis B, one type of influenza vaccine (Flublok), acellular pertussis (the pertussis vaccine used in the United States), and one type of typhoid vaccine.

There are two ways to create a subunit vaccine. Both methods are difficult and costly. First, researchers must identify the pathogen's antigenic surface proteins. Next, they must determine which proteins create the strongest immune response. Once these proteins have been identified, one way to obtain them is to grow the pathogen large quantities in the laboratory. The whole pathogen is then treated with chemicals to break up the antigens on its surface, after which they can be purified for use in a vaccine.

A second way to make a subunit vaccine is through genetic engineering. This is possible because advances in biotechnology have reduced the time and cost of sequencing genomes and created new gene-splicing tools. Subunit vaccines made through genetic engineering are called recombinant subunit vaccines because genetic material from the pathogen is combined with genetic material of a nonpathogenic organism that then produces the desired antigens.

To make a recombinant subunit vaccine, scientists first identify the genetic material (DNA or RNA) of the pathogen that codes for the pathogen's antigenic proteins. Using gene-splicing enzymes, this material is snipped out of the pathogen and inserted into the genetic material of a harmless organism such as a yeast cell. The spliced-in bit of genetic information then directs the host cells to make surface antigens identical to that of the pathogen from which it was taken. The antigens that are produced can be separated and purified for use in a vaccine.

A third version of subunit vaccine called a recombinant vector vaccine is under development. Making this vaccine is similar to making a recombinant subunit vaccine described earlier. Some of the genetic material of a pathogen is spliced into the genetic material of a host organism, which is either a harmless virus or an attenuated bacterium. The difference between a recombinant subunit vaccine and a recombinant vector vaccine is that rather than growing the host organism and harvesting the antigenic proteins it produces, the whole host organism (which is now called a vector) is injected into a human. The vector does not negatively affect human health, but as it reproduces, it makes the antigenic proteins coded for by the pathogen's genetic material. The immune system reacts to these antigenic proteins and forms antibodies and memory cells. In a sense, the body becomes its own vaccine factory.

Like other subunit vaccines, recombinant vector vaccines cannot cause illness because only part of the pathogen is reproduced. Vector vaccines are more stable and less temperature sensitive than live attenuated vaccines, are faster to manufacture, cost less, and are easier to alter. Disadvantages include the risk of inappropriate gene expression or mutation of the pathogen's DNA, difficulties in scaling production to commercial levels, and public skepticism about the safety of genetic engineering. As of mid-2018, no recombinant vector vaccines were licensed for human use in the United States, although several recombinant vector veterinary vaccines, including a West Nile vaccine for horses, had been approved.

POLYSACCHARIDE AND CONJUGATE VACCINES

Some disease-causing bacteria are encased in a polysaccharide (complex sugar) capsule that helps them escape detection by immune system cells. Polysaccharide vaccines are a type of subunit vaccine made from pieces of this capsule; the whole organism is not used. The drawback to polysaccharide vaccines is that immune system does not respond to polysaccharide antigens as strongly as it does to protein antigens. Response is especially poor in children under two years old. Repeated doses of polysaccharide vaccines do not produce additional or prolonged immunity as they do with inactivated/killed vaccines. Versions of pneumococcal, meningococcal, and typhoid vaccines are polysaccharide vaccines.

Conjugate vaccines were developed in the late 1980s to overcome the problem of inadequate immune response to polysaccharide vaccines. To make a conjugate vaccine, the desired part of the polysaccharide capsule is isolated and purified, and then a harmless protein is chemically attached to the piece of capsule. The protein boosts immune system response and makes the vaccine more effective in creating immunological memory, especially in young children. The first conjugate vaccine was *Haemophilus influenzae* type b (Hib). As of 2018, pneumococcal and meningococcal conjugate vaccines (MCV) are also in use. Table 3.1 summarizes the types of vaccines and the way in which the antigenic component for each type of vaccine is obtained.

Table 3.1 Production of Antigenic Components

Vaccine Type	Vaccines	How Immunologic Component Is Produced
Live attenuated viral vaccines	Adenovirus, measles, mumps, oral polio vaccine,[†] rotavirus, rubella, smallpox, yellow fever, varicella, and zoster	Grown in a hostile environment to force mutations that reduce reproductive capacity in humans
Live attenuated bacterial vaccines	Bacille Calmette-Guérin vaccine (BCG), cholera, plague, and one form of typhoid vaccine; these vaccines are not routinely used in the United States	Grown in a hostile environment to force mutations that reduce reproductive capacity in humans
Inactivated or killed vaccines	Hepatitis A, inactivated influenza vaccine, Japanese encephalitis, inactivated polio vaccine, and rabies and whole cell pertussis[†]	Inactivated/killed with chemicals or heat
Toxoid vaccines	Diphtheria and tetanus	Purified toxin deactivated with chemicals or heat
Subunit vaccines	Anthrax, hepatitis B, HPV, influenza (Flublok), acellular pertussis, one type of typhoid vaccine., and Lyme disease[†]	Identification and isolation of surface antigens or production of surface antigens by genetic engineering (recombinant vaccines)
Polysaccharide vaccines	Some versions of meningococcal, pneumococcal, and typhoid vaccines	Identification and isolation of surface antigens on polysaccharide coat
Conjugate vaccines	*Haemophilus influenzae* type b (Hib), some versions of meningococcal and pneumococcal vaccines	Protein attached to polysaccharide coat to increase antigen response

† No longer used in the United States.

POLYVALENT VACCINES

Some pathogens have diversified into multiple strains or subspecies. Although these strains are closely related, their surface antigens are slightly different. Polyvalent vaccines contain the antigens of several subspecies of a pathogen to broaden the immunity the vaccine creates. For example, influenza vaccine contains antigens against three or four different strains of influenza depending on the formulation. Other examples of polyvalent vaccines are those against human papillomavirus (HPV), meningococcal bacteria, pneumococcal bacteria, and polio.

Polyvalent vaccines can be made in any of the ways described earlier. They provide more extensive immunity without requiring additional shots, although immunity may not develop as strongly or as rapidly as it would with a monovalent vaccine. Protection against more strains of a pathogen outweighs this disadvantage.

COMBINATION VACCINES

Combination vaccines protect against two or more diseases in a single shot. Two combination vaccines, diphtheria, tetanus, and acellular pertussis (DTaP) and mumps, measles, and rubella (MMR) have been used for many years. Newer combinations include Hib and hepatitis B; hepatitis A and hepatitis B; MMR and varicella (chickenpox); DTaP and IPV; DTaP, IPV, and hepatitis B; DTaP and hepatitis B; and DTaP, IPV, and Hib. Combination vaccine administration schedules differ from those of single vaccines.

The advantages of combination vaccines are that they require fewer shots and health care visits. They reduce shipping and storage costs and provide a faster path to full vaccination. In developing countries, combination vaccines are especially valuable because they make it easier for children with limited access to health care to become fully vaccinated.

Although combination vaccines are tested to assure the components do not interfere with each other, many vaccine-skeptic parents worry that the presence of so many antigens may overstress a child's immune system. These parents often request that vaccines be given separately for each disease and with longer intervals between shots. This is not always possible. For example, there is no single vaccine against measles or whooping cough (pertussis) licensed in the United States. Controversy about combination vaccines is addressed in the second part of this book in Chapter 11.

VACCINE COMPONENTS

A vaccine is more than a collection of antigens. Other substances must be added to stabilize the vaccine for transport and storage, protect against contamination by other organisms, assure the proper concentration of antigens, and in some cases boost the effectiveness of the antigens. In addition, trace amounts of materials used to grow, attenuate, inactivate/kill pathogens, or prepare subunit antigens may remain in the vaccine. A list of all components of each vaccine can be found at https://vaccines.procon.org/view.resource.php?resourceID=005206 or in Section 11 (Description) of the vaccine package insert. Inserts are available online at www.immunize.org/packageinserts.

Suspending Fluid

Suspending fluid is the liquid in which all the components of a vaccine are dissolved. Suspending fluid is either sterile water, saline (salt water), or liquid containing buffering proteins. Some vaccines are shipped as ready-to-use liquids. Others (e.g., measles, yellow fever, rabies, BCG) are too unstable to be shipped in their suspending fluid. These vaccines are processed into a freeze-dried powder that contains the antigen. Before use, they are reconstituted with a diluent specific to each vaccine that contains the exact amount of stabilizers, preservatives, and sterile suspending fluid for each vaccine. Once the diluent is added, the vaccine must be used within a few hours.

Stabilizers

Stabilizers help protect vaccines during the freeze-drying process, shield them against changes in temperature, and maintain their potency. Some stabilizers are sugars and proteins found in many foods and drugs. Examples are the sugars lactose and sucrose; sorbitol, which is another common sweetener; monosodium glutamate, a flavor enhancer used in foods; and gelatin. Less familiar chemicals such as phosphate buffers and magnesium sulfate may also be added to adjust the pH (acidity or alkalinity) of the solution. Human albumin, a protein found in blood, can also be used as a stabilizer.

Preservatives

Preservatives are antiseptic chemicals used to kill bacteria and fungi. The use of preservatives in vaccines developed in the 1920s after incidents where people died as the result of contamination of a vaccine with tetanus, the spores of which are common in soil and dust. Antibiotics had not yet been discovered, so very low doses of antiseptic chemicals were added to control contamination. Four chemical preservatives are licensed for use in vaccines in the United States in 2018: phenol, 2-phenoxyethanol, thimerosal, and benzethonium chloride. Benzethonium chloride is used only in anthrax vaccine, which is reserved almost exclusively for military use.

Phenol, also called carbolic acid, is an antiseptic that was used in carbolic soap until the 1970s and today is found in many drugs, cosmetics, and sunscreens. Phenol is also made by the body and is excreted in urine. The preservative 2-phenoxyethanol is widely used in perfumes, cosmetics, and insecticides. It is effective in killing bacteria and yeasts.

Thimerosal has been the most controversial preservative used in vaccines because of its mercury content. It was added to vaccines from the 1940s to 2001, at which time it was eliminated as a preservative from all vaccines routinely used in the United States for children under age six years except for influenza vaccine. A thimerosal-free version of influenza vaccine is now available. Thimerosal is still included in some vaccines shipped in multidose vials for use outside the United States. It is added to multi-dose vials because of the potential for contamination when injection needles are dipped into the vial to extract a dose of vaccine for use. Anti-vaccination advocates have claimed that thimerosal in vaccines caused autism, attention deficit hyperactivity disorder, and other neuropsychological disorders despite many studies showing there is no link between thimerosal and these disorders. This controversy is discussed in Chapter 10.

Antibiotics

In some vaccines, small amounts of antibiotics are used to prevent bacterial and fungal contamination. Because a significant number of people are allergic to penicillins, cephalosporins, and sulfa drugs, these antibiotics are not used in vaccines. Instead, neomycin, polymyxin B, streptomycin, and gentamicin, all antibiotics that are less likely to cause an allergic reaction, are used for contamination control.

Vaccines against measles, mumps, rubella, chickenpox, shingles, rabies, diphtheria, pertussis, tetanus, hepatitis A, hepatitis B, and some influenza vaccines contain antibiotics, as do combination vaccines against these diseases. Neomycin is the most common used. The amount per dose is very small, ranging from 0.15 mg of neomycin in rabies vaccine to less than 0.000000004 mg of neomycin in some formulations of DTaP.

Adjuvants

The word "adjuvant" comes from the Latin word *adjuvaere,* meaning "to help." Adjuvants are chemicals added to some vaccines to boost the effectiveness of the antigenic component. This allows immunity to develop using a lower concentration of antigen or with fewer doses of vaccine. Diphtheria and tetanus vaccines developed in the 1930s were the first to contain adjuvants.

As of 2018, only two types of adjuvants had been approved in the United States. Aluminum in the form of aluminum hydroxide, aluminum phosphate, or potassium aluminum sulfate (also called alum) is used in DTaP and Tdap (tetanus, diphtheria, and pertussis), hepatitis A, hepatitis B,

Hib, some types of HPV, one form of trivalent influenza vaccine, and pneumococcal vaccines. The amount of aluminum in vaccines is limited to 0.85–1.25 mg per dose, whereas the average American adult has a median intake of 24 mg of aluminum daily in drinking water, food, and pharmaceutical drugs such as antacids.

Monophosphoryl lipid A, a fat-like compound isolated from the cell wall of a bacterium, was approved for use as an adjuvant in 2009. It is used in combination with aluminum hydroxide in the HPV vaccine Cervarix. The controversy surrounding the safety of adjuvants is discussed in Chapter 9.

The mechanism by which adjuvants boost immune response is not completely understood. Some researchers believe they help to hold the antigen at the injection site, allowing slower but longer stimulation of immune system cells. Alternately, they may stimulate antigens to clump and form large complexes that are more easily engulfed by antigen-presenting cells.

Production Residues

Production residues are traces amounts of materials used during the making of a vaccine. These residues vary depending on the vaccine and the manufacturing process. For example, formalin is used to neutralize the toxin in the toxoid vaccines against diphtheria and tetanus and to inactivate viruses so that they cannot cause disease. Formalin is removed during the production process, but tiny amounts remain in vaccines such as IPV, hepatitis A, rabies, diphtheria, and tetanus. The body naturally produces far greater amounts of formalin during normal metabolic functioning than are contained in a dose of vaccine. Both naturally produced formalin and vaccine-introduced formalin are broken down and excreted from the body.

Some live attenuated viruses such as influenza, measles, and yellow fever are grown in chicken eggs. When the viruses are harvested, small amounts of egg protein remain in these vaccines, as well as in the combination vaccines MMR and MMRV (MMR plus varicella). This can be of concern to people who have egg allergies (about 1% of young children). The amount of egg protein in MMR and MMRV is tiny and has not been shown to cause an allergic reaction. However, reactions in people allergic to eggs have been reported with influenza and yellow fever vaccine. A recombinant influenza vaccine that contains no egg residue can be used to safely vaccinate people with egg allergy.

Hepatitis B vaccine is subunit vaccine made using baker's yeast. Traces of yeast remain in the vaccine whether it is given alone or in a combination vaccine. One version HPV vaccine (Gardasil) also contains yeast. This can be of concern to individuals with a yeast allergy.

Because viruses cannot reproduce on their own, they need to be grown in a culture containing live cells. Varicella, zoster, rubella, hepatitis A, and one version of the rabies vaccine all are made using cultures containing either human or animal cells. Although trace proteins from these cells may remain after the viruses are purified, they do not appear to cause adverse reactions.

VACCINE ADMINISTRATION

Just as not all vaccines contain the same components, not all vaccines are administered in the same way. The choice of vaccine and the way it is given depend on the vaccine's purpose, how it is transported through the body, which method of administration produces the fewest adverse events, and its ease of use. Often different versions of a vaccine are made to meet the needs of specific populations. Vaccines may be manufactured in different strengths or with different dosage regimens for different age groups.

- Intramuscular (IM) injection is the most common route of administration. IM vaccines include anthrax, diphtheria, hepatitis A, hepatitis B, Hib, HPV, influenza (IIV and RIV), IPV, Japanese encephalitis, MCV, pertussis, pneumococcal, rabies, tetanus, DTaP, and most combination vaccines except MMR and MMRV. The site of injection depends on age. Children under two years old are given injections in the thigh muscle, while older children and adults normally are injected in an arm muscle.
- Subcutaneous injections (SC) place the vaccine below the skin but above the muscle. Meningococcal polysaccharide, varicella, zoster (shingles), and yellow fever, along with combination vaccines MMR and MMRV are given this way.
- Oral administration is by mouth. Vaccines that affect pathogens that grow in the digestive system are usually given this way. Adenovirus, cholera, OPV, and rotavirus vaccines are delivered orally.
- Intradermal administration (ID) is the least common route of administration. It involves injecting the vaccine with a sterile needle under only the top layer of skin. ID is the most difficult route of administration for most health care practitioners. BCG (tuberculosis) vaccine is always given ID, and one form of the influenza vaccine (Fluzone intradermal) can be given this way, although IM influenza immunization is much more common.

To summarize, the Food and Drug Administration regulates vaccine development and production under federal laws. In creating a new vaccine, developers must consider the characteristics of the pathogen, strength of immune response, appropriate dosage, and seriousness of undesirable side effects along with issues such as cost, ease of production, transport, storage, ease of use, and the size of the potential market.

Vaccines are made in various ways. Live attenuated vaccines contain live but weakened viruses. Inactivated/killed vaccines contain whole pathogens that are inactive/dead and are incapable of causing disease. Subunit vaccines contain only antigens from the pathogen, not the whole organism. They can be made by growing the pathogen and extracting the antigens or by genetic engineering techniques. Polysaccharide and conjugate vaccines are special types of subunit vaccines for pathogens that are encased in a polysaccharide coat. Polyvalent vaccines protect against more than one strain of a pathogen. Combination vaccines protect against more than one disease in a single shot.

The antigen is the active part of a vaccine, but vaccines also contain some or all of the following: suspending fluid, antibiotics, preservatives, and adjuvants. These components serve to protect the purity of the vaccine, extend shelf life, and boost effectiveness. Production residues are trace amounts of chemicals and cells that are used in making the vaccine.

Vaccines against the same disease can be made in more than one form, strength, or combination. Vaccines can be administered intramuscularly (most common), subcutaneously, orally, or intradermally (least common), depending on the purpose of the vaccine and the population being vaccinated.

CHAPTER 4

Regulation of Vaccines

Vaccines are regulated by law from early development through testing, manufacturing, distribution, storage, and disposal. In the United States, the federal government is responsible for these aspects of regulation. The individual states are responsible for the laws that control who must be vaccinated and what exemptions are permitted. Other countries have their own regulations, and the World Health Organization has a certification process used by many developing countries. The following information applies to oversight in the United States.

EARLY REGULATION

The first federal attempt to regulate vaccines was made when Congress passed the National Vaccine Act of 1813 to encourage vaccination. The purpose of the Act was to appoint a national vaccine agent to preserve and distribute a national source of uncontaminated smallpox vaccine. Dr. James Smith, a Baltimore physician active in getting the bill passed, was appointed the first vaccine agent. He was charged with developing the policies of the National Vaccine Agency. As an incentive to encourage vaccine distribution, postage was not charged on any mail that contained smallpox vaccine.

Smith ran into funding problems almost immediately. States were willing to have their residents vaccinated, but they did not want to pay for a federal vaccine program. Residents either could not afford the vaccine or did not feel they should have to pay for it. A major objection was the claim that Congress had given Smith an unfair monopoly on smallpox vaccine.

Smith struggled with various funding schemes until 1822 when a small-pox epidemic started by his vaccine killed 10 people in Tarboro, North Carolina. Smith claimed that Dr. John Ward, who requested the vaccine, had administered it improperly. Ward claimed the vaccine was bad. The issue was escalated to the national level by Representative Hutchins Burton who was running for (and was later elected) governor of North Carolina. In May 1822, Congress found it politically expedient to repeal the National Vaccine Act without ever hearing testimony from Ward. This ended the first attempt to regulate vaccines at the national level.

The federal government did nothing to regulate vaccines for the next 80 years, but in 1902, the death in St. Louis of 13 children from diphtheria antitoxin contaminated with tetanus stimulated Congress to pass the Biologics Control Act. This Act required manufacturers of antitoxins, serums, and vaccines to be inspected and licensed annually. A qualified scientist had to oversee production, and labels were required to include the name of the product, expiration date, and manufacturer contact information. Responsibility for enforcement was given to the Laboratory of Hygiene, which later became the National Institutes of Health (NIH). In 1988, responsibility for regulation of biologic products was transferred to the Center for Biologics Evaluation and Research within the Food and Drug Administration (FDA), where it remains today.

In 1906, Upton Sinclair's book, *The Jungle,* exposed appalling unsanitary conditions in the meatpacking industry. Public reaction to the book resulted in the passage of the Pure Food and Drug Act. The Act did not specifically address vaccines, but it prohibited the manufacture, sale, or transportation of all adulterated, mislabeled, or poisonous foods, drugs, medicines, and liquors. The Act also required all active ingredients and those designated as dangerous or addictive (e.g., morphine, cocaine, alcohol) to appear on the label. Fines could be assessed for noncompliance, but the real power of the Act was a provision that allowed seizure and destruction of nonconforming products. Inspection and enforcement powers were given to the Bureau of Chemistry, which became part of the FDA in 1930.

The Pure Food and Drug Act was replaced by the Federal Food, Drug, and Cosmetic Act of 1938. This Act has been amended many times since its passage to keep up with changing demands of the public and new technologies. For example, the 1962 the Kefauver Harris Amendment, also known as the Drug Efficacy Amendment, required drug manufacturers to perform studies to prove that a new drug was safe and effective before it was licensed. The amendment also required drug advertising to include accurate information on potential side effects, which is why today when drugs are advertised on television or in print, they include a long list of potential adverse events. These three Acts remain the backbone of regulation in the United States for the development of all drugs including vaccines.

Vaccine Development Requirements

Development of a vaccine begins with basic scientific research usually conducted in a university, medical center laboratory, or government-supported laboratory. Basic research involves studying the genetics and metabolism of the pathogen, identifying and isolating antigens, testing potential host cells, and studying mechanisms by which the immune system responds to the antigen. The process is international and incremental, with different groups of researchers working on the same problem from several angles and publishing their work in scientific journals where other scientists can evaluate it. Failure is more common than success.

Early Challenges

Once a promising antigen has been identified and isolated, the cost of research often shifts to a pharmaceutical company, which supports both outside and in-house research. The antigen must be adequately purified before testing. Testing usually begins on small rodents, often ferrets. Researchers look to see if the animal produces antibodies when challenged by the antigen. If small animal results look promising, the antigen is tested on larger animals whose biology is more like humans. Animal testing also provides insight into the strength and duration of immunity.

Phase I Clinical Trials

If the results of animal research show a new vaccine has promise, a sponsor is required to file an Investigational New Drug (IND) application with the FDA. Sponsors usually are pharmaceutical companies. For a drug to receive IND approval, proof that it is reasonably safe and has potential for commercial development must be presented. Approval of the IND allows a drug or biological product to be shipped across state lines to outside investigators, something necessary for continued testing.

Human testing begins with Phase I clinical trials. All clinical trials are subject to FDA regulation and oversight and use only volunteers. Phase I trials involve only a small number of volunteers—usually somewhere between 30 and 50. The goal of Phase I is to answer two questions: Is the vaccine safe? Does the vaccine produce the expected immune response? The test vaccine must contain the adjuvants, preservatives, and stabilizers that will be in the final product. It takes years and millions of dollars to reach Phase I trials. The trial itself usually takes one to two years to complete.

Phase II Clinical Trials

If the results from Phase I trials are favorable, the vaccine enters Phase II trials. The goal of Phase II is to determine the correct dosage of the vaccine and to study its safety in a larger population. Up to this point, only a small amount of vaccine was needed, but Phase II trials require vaccine for a minimum of several hundred volunteers, so while Phase I trials are under way, researchers study ways to scale up production.

One FDA requirement is that vaccine used in Phase II trials must be manufactured in the building where the final vaccine will be made. This often requires building new facilities or special production and storage rooms, massive amounts of equipment, and a significant financial commitment by the manufacturer before it knows whether the vaccine will ever be licensed for sale. The company must also show how the newly manufactured vaccine will be tested and prove that the tests used produce reliable, reproducible results. Even vaccines that do well in Phase I testing may be abandoned because the manufacturer decides that its return on investment will be too low to justify the increased costs of moving on to Phase II. Phase II trials can take as few as two years but preparing for this phase usually takes much longer.

Phase III Clinical Trials

Phase III trials are large-scale controlled field tests necessary before a vaccine is licensed. In most cases, they are double-blind trials, meaning that neither the volunteers nor the health care workers running the trial know whether the individual receives the vaccine (the experimental group) or a placebo (the control group). In some cases, such as with Ebola vaccine, giving a placebo to people who could contract a fatal disease is considered unethical, and an alternate form of evaluation called ring vaccination is used to determine the vaccine's effectiveness.

Phase III trials usually involve thousands of people because the number of volunteers must be great enough to determine statistical differences between experimental and control groups. Volunteers must meet certain age and health requirements in keeping with the target population for the vaccine. At this point, the vaccine is manufactured almost as it would be if it were licensed. Its strength, contents, directions for distribution, storage, administration, expiration date, and labeling are all in place. Tests have been certified to assure the purity and effectiveness of every batch of vaccine. Other tests have been developed to reliably determine the volunteers' response to the vaccine, and procedures are in place to record adverse events and statistically compare control and experimental groups. Test sites are monitored and visited by representatives of the FDA, and reams of data are collected.

Phase III trials usually last about four years, depending on how common the disease is and how easy it is to recruit volunteers. It then takes the company another 18 months to 2 years to review the data and prepare a biologics license application for the FDA. Once the application is received, the FDA reviews trial data, inspects the manufacturing facility, and reviews the labeling, all of which can take another year before the vaccine is licensed and can be sold to the public.

THE NATIONAL CHILDHOOD VACCINE INJURY ACT

The federal government continues to remain involved in vaccine regulation after licensure. In 1979, three-month-old Kevin Toner was inoculated with DPT (diphtheria, pertussis, and tetanus) vaccine and developed a rare infection of the spinal cord called transverse myelitis that left him permanently paralyzed below the waist. His parents sued the vaccine manufacturer, Lederle Laboratories, claiming that the pertussis component of the vaccine had caused Kevin's paralysis.

The pertussis vaccine had been licensed since the 1940s, and in almost 40 years, no increase above the background rate of spinal cord inflammation had been observed in vaccinated children. Nevertheless, the jury that heard *Toner v. Lederle Laboratories* awarded Kevin Toner's parents $1.13 million (equivalent to $4.4 million in 2018 dollars). The jury based the award not on a connection between DPT vaccine and the child's injury but on the plaintiff's argument that the manufacturer was negligent because it could have made a safer vaccine. The case was appealed, but the Idaho Supreme Court upheld the award.

The verdict against Lederle Laboratories sent shock waves through the vaccine industry for two reasons. First, the manufacturer was found negligent in the absence of a scientific connection between its product and the child's injury. Second, the award was far larger than anyone expected. In 1979, the gross annual sales of DPT vaccine were about $2 million and total gross sales of all vaccines were only about $7 million. A few awards the size of *Toner v. Lederle Laboratories* could wipe out a company, especially a smaller one whose main products were vaccines. Many pharmaceutical companies had already gotten out of the vaccine business. Fear of financial ruin accelerated this trend. After the *Toner v. Lederle Laboratories* decision, companies that continued to make vaccines drastically raised their prices. From 1980 to 1986, the cost of a single dose of DPT vaccine rose from $0.19 to $12.00. At this point, the federal government stepped in to stabilize the vaccine industry.

In 1986, competing interest groups were lobbying Congress for changes in the vaccine industry. Parents wanted a way to receive speedy compensation for vaccine-related injuries without going through lengthy civil trials and appeals. Vaccine manufacturers needed protection from outsized financial awards. Health care providers sought protection against being sued, as did manufacturers and distributors. The government wanted to assure the supply of vaccines would remain adequate and affordable to protect public health. Out of these competing interests came the federal National Childhood Vaccine Injury Act (NCVIA).

The NCVIA created the National Vaccine Program Office to coordinate all immunization-related activities across multiple agencies such as the FDA, the Centers for Disease Control and Prevention (CDC), the NIH, and the Department of Health and Human Services (DHHS). The Act requires anyone who administers a vaccine to provide the person being inoculated or that person's parent or guardian with a CDC-approved vaccine information statement that describes the disease being immunized against and the benefits and risks of the vaccine. Current versions of these statements can be accessed at https://www.cdc.gov/vaccines/hcp/vis. NCVIA also established the Vaccine Adverse Event Reporting System (VAERS) and the Vaccine Injury Compensation Program (VICP).

THE VACCINE ADVERSE EVENT REPORTING SYSTEM

The VAERS is a postlicensing vaccine safety surveillance system sponsored by the CDC and the FDA. The purpose of VAERS is to

- detect new or rare adverse events that may have gone undetected during clinical trials;
- monitor increases in known adverse events;
- determine risk factors that make some individuals more susceptible to adverse events;
- identify vaccine lots associated with increased adverse events; and
- assess the ongoing safety of newly licensed vaccines.

Health care providers are required to report certain serious adverse events that appear within a specified period after vaccination. However, any person may voluntarily report any type of adverse event to VAERS online or by mail. Adverse events are any undesirable experience that occurs soon after inoculation. The reporting party does not have to prove that the vaccine caused the adverse event as long as the report is made in good faith.

In 2015, VAERS received 41,335 adverse event reports. The highest percentage was for people ages 44–61, followed by people ages 17–44. This is surprising given that the greatest number of vaccines are given to children. About 85 percent of reported adverse events were mild. The staff at VAERS follows up by asking for additional medical information on serious events to help determine if the vaccine may have caused the reported incident.

OTHER POSTLICENSURE SURVEILLANCE

In addition to VAERS, which depends on voluntary reporting, other government organizations also perform proactive postlicensure surveillance. The Vaccine Safety Data Link receives information from health care providers for about nine million patients (roughly 3 percent of the population) each year. Using this information, the frequency of certain disorders in unvaccinated children can be compared to the frequency of these same disorders in vaccinated children. The rate in unvaccinated children becomes the background rate for the disorder. If the frequency of the disorder in vaccinated children rises above the background rate, the possibility that the vaccine is contributing to the disorder must be evaluated.

The Clinical Immunization Safety Assessment Project established in 2001 in partnership with the CDC is a network of eight nationally recognized medical centers and vaccine experts. Its function is to study risk factors in special populations, develop strategies for identifying individuals at higher risk for adverse effects from vaccination, develop preventative strategies, and serve as a resource for clinicians making immunization decisions.

The Post-Licensure Rapid Immunization Safety Monitoring (PRISM) system established in 2009 under the direction of the FDA is the largest postlicensing vaccine safety surveillance program in the United States. Through electronic databases, it has access to historical information for over 100 million people. PRISM links databases from national health insurance plans and state immunization registries to perform statistical

analyses that when combined with information from voluntary reporting
of adverse events to VAERS allow the detection of the rare adverse effects.

NATIONAL VACCINE INJURY COMPENSATION PROGRAM

The VICP began in October 1988 and continues today. The VICP is a
government program that assumes financial risk for proven vaccine injures.
It operates outside the civil court system and is financed by an excise tax on
vaccines. The VICP has multiple goals:

- It protects vaccine manufacturers from catastrophic financial loss
  resulting from liability lawsuits alleging injury caused by vaccines.
  This encourages pharmaceutical companies to stay in the vaccine
  business and helps to stabilize the cost of vaccines.
- It helps assure the government that an adequate supply of vaccine
  will remain available to protect public health.
- The program provides a faster and less expensive way for vaccine-
  injured individuals to receive compensation than bringing a liability
  case to civil court.

Despite these advantages, the existence of this program is proof for some
anti-vaccinationists that the government knows vaccines are unsafe and
is colluding with pharmaceutical companies to hide the evidence (see
Chapter 13).

Vaccines covered by the VICP must be on the CDC list of recommended vaccines for routine administration to children, subject to excise
tax by federal law, and be added to the VICP by the Secretary of Health
and Human Services. Newly licensed vaccines that fall into the same category as an already covered vaccine are automatically covered. As of 2018,
the covered vaccines were diphtheria, tetanus, pertussis, *Haemophilus
influenzae* type b (Hib), hepatitis A, hepatitis B, human papillomavirus,
seasonal influenza, measles, mumps, rubella, meningococcal, polio, pneumococcal conjugate, rotavirus, and varicella in any combination such as
DTaP or MMRV. Only specific vaccine injuries listed in the Vaccine Injury
Table (VIT) are normally compensated even for VICP-listed vaccines. The
complete table can be located through https://www.hrsa.gov/vaccine-com
pensation/index.html.

Disabilities or injuries caused by adulterants or contaminants in a vaccine are also not covered under the VICP, although they can be the basis
for a civil suit against the manufacturer.

How the VICP Works

A person of any age, the parent or legal guardian of a child, or the legal representative of the estate of a deceased person who believes the individual was harmed by a covered vaccine can make a claim under the VICP within a defined time frame. The cost of filing a claim as of 2018 was $400. Representation by an attorney is not required; however, most petitioners use an attorney who specializes in vaccine injuries to meet the highly specific rules and deadlines for filing. Under most circumstances, the VICP will pay attorney fees related to a claim even if the petitioner's request for compensation is denied.

Petitioners filing for damages must produce an abundance of medical records of treatments both before and after vaccination to justify their claim. Prevaccination records include prenatal records for the mother if a young child is the petitioner, hospital records for the delivery and newborn hospital stay, a birth certificate, and all additional medical records such as doctor visits and laboratory work done outside the hospital prior to vaccination.

Postvaccination records include all medical records for emergency treatment, hospital admissions, medications, laboratory reports, evaluations, and outpatient treatment that occurred. Depending on the type of injury, school records and educational and psychological evaluations may be required to determine the validity and extent of damage. In the case of death, a death certificate and autopsy (if done) are required. When possible, the vaccine lot number and manufacturer are requested.

After analysis by attorneys at the Department of Justice and medical experts at the DHHS, a report goes to Federal Claims Court where a judge appoints a Special Master. The Special Master is an independent attorney who evaluates the claim and decides whether it should be paid and, if so, the amount of compensation. The petitioner can accept or reject the Special Master's decision. If the petitioner rejects the decision, the case can be appealed first to a judge in the Federal Claims Court, then to the U.S. Court of Appeals, and finally to the U.S. Supreme Court, but once the appeals process is started, the petitioner cannot change his or her mind and accept a Special Master's offer of compensation.

Unless there are highly unusual circumstances, vaccine injuries are compensated only when they

- are listed in the VIT;
- develop within the designated time frame;
- are adequately documented; and
- cannot be shown to have another cause.

For conditions not listed in the VIT or that that develop outside the defined period, the burden falls on the petitioner to prove that a cause-and-effect relationship exists between the vaccine and the injury. The vaccine court procedure is complicated, but few claims go through the complete process described here. According to the DHHS, 80 percent of cases are settled through negotiation between the involved parties rather than by the Special Master. Extensive information on the VICP can be found at https://www.hrsa.gov/vaccine-compensation/data/index.html.

State Regulations

The United States does not have national vaccination requirements for its citizens nor are there any entry vaccination requirements for tourists and short-term visitors. The only national vaccination requirements apply to immigrants and people who want to adjust their status to that of a permanent resident. To obtain an immigrant visa or permanent residency, a person must have proof of receiving all age-appropriate vaccines recommended by the Advisory Committee for Immunization Practices. Beyond this, each state determines which vaccines are required for its citizens.

As of 2018, all 50 states and the District of Columbia required children entering public school to be vaccinated against diphtheria, tetanus, pertussis, polio, measles, and rubella. All but Iowa required vaccination against mumps. Most states also required vaccination against chickenpox and hepatitis B. State law also determines if these requirements apply to private schools or daycare centers. Private employers may require vaccinations for certain health care providers, first responders, and people at high risk for contracting a vaccine-preventable disease such as those working with a pathogen in the laboratory.

All 50 states and the District of Columbia allow medical exemptions from vaccination. Religious exemptions are allowed in 47 states, and 17 states permit personal belief exemptions. More information about state vaccination laws and exemptions can be found at https://www.cdc.gov/phlp/publica tions/topic/vaccinations.html. Chapter 12 discusses these legal requirements and exemptions more extensively.

In conclusion, in the United States, there are two aspects to vaccine regulation. The development, testing, licensing, manufacturing, storage, transport, and disposal of vaccines are regulated at the national level. The federal government has set up the VICP to compensate individuals provably damaged by a vaccine. The program operates outside the regular court system.

Requirements concerning who must be vaccinated and against which vaccine-preventable disease are determined by state law and vary from state to state. State vaccination laws apply primarily to children in public school, private school, and daycare. Adult daycare and health care workers may also be affected by mandatory vaccination laws. All states allow medical exemptions from vaccination. Most states allow religious exemptions, but less than half permit personal belief exemptions.

CHAPTER 5

Vaccines and the Diseases They Prevent

There is no uniform procedure for giving vaccines. Each one has a unique protocol that specifies the route of administration, dosage, age for inoculation, required interval between inoculations, precautions, and restrictions on the population to be vaccinated. Every year, the Centers for Disease Control and Prevention (CDC) releases a recommended immunization schedule based on a review of vaccine data by the Advisory Committee on Immunization Practices (ACIP). ACIP members are vaccine experts. Protocols are arrived at after extensive testing and data analysis from clinical trials. Nevertheless, once a vaccine is in widespread use, recommendations can change based on information collected from postlicensure data and physicians' experience with their patients.

The World Health Organization (WHO) also makes recommendations to strengthen and extend coverage of routine vaccinations worldwide as part of its Global Vaccine Action Plan. The WHO recommendations are developed by vaccine experts who consider the same criteria as ACIP, but the WHO recommendations may differ based on the needs and limitations of various national immunization programs and the prevalence of disease in different parts of the world.

All major medical organizations strongly endorse the CDC-recommended schedule, but it is often challenged by vaccine skeptics who claim that ACIP is biased on the side of the pharmaceutical companies whose goal is to profit from selling as many vaccines as possible. In response to this concern, a few pediatricians have created their own untested alternate vaccination schedule. This controversy is discussed in Chapter 11.

Vaccines Routinely Used in the United States

The information on vaccines in this section is based on the CDC-recommended standard vaccination schedule for 2018 for healthy Americans. Appropriate vaccine administration for certain subpopulations may vary at the discretion of the individual's physician. Vaccines are listed alphabetically, not by age of administration.

Diphtheria, Tetanus, and Pertussis

Immunization against diphtheria, tetanus (lockjaw), and pertussis (whooping cough) is given as a combination vaccine. Diphtheria, tetanus, and acellular pertussis (DTaP) is the combination used in the United States for children younger than age seven years. Acellular pertussis is a subunit vaccine that contains only antigens from the pertussis pathogen. It causes fewer adverse effects than the killed whole-cell pertussis vaccine (DPT or DTwP) used earlier. Whole-cell pertussis vaccine is still used internationally. Some recent studies suggest that it provides longer-lasting immunity than DTaP.

DT is an alternative for children who cannot tolerate any pertussis vaccine. Less frequently used is a four-combination vaccine that immunizes against diphtheria, tetanus, pertussis, and polio (Kinrix) and a five-combination vaccine against hepatitis B, diphtheria, tetanus, pertussis, and polio (Pediarix). These combination vaccines have administration schedules and age restrictions that differ from DTaP and DT.

A slightly different formulation called Tdap (lower case d and p indicate reduced-strength doses) is used for children over age seven and adults. Td is a booster shot given to adults every 10 years because childhood immunization does not provide lifelong immunity.

Diphtheria

Symptoms of diphtheria are caused by a toxin released by the bacterium *Corynebacterium diphtheriae*. Diphtheria begins with symptoms similar to the common cold. However, unlike cold viruses, C. *diphtheriae* bacteria stick to the cells lining the airways. As toxin is released, it damages these cells. Soon, a membrane forms made of dead blood cells and fibrin, a blood-clotting protein. The membrane can completely block the airway, resulting in death by asphyxiation.

In the mid-1920s, before an effective diphtheria vaccine became widely available, the disease infected about 200,000 people annually with a death rate as high as 20 percent in children less than five years old. Today, very few cases of diphtheria occur in the United States, usually among the homeless, people who were incompletely immunized, Native Americans, and travelers from regions where the disease is active. Outbreaks in the early 2000s in the Baltic States, Eastern Europe, and sub-Saharan Africa killed more than 5,000 people. In 2016, 35 countries reported diphtheria cases. A person who is completely immunized and symptom-free can be a carrier for the disease and transmit it to someone who does not have immunity.

Tetanus

Tetanus is caused by a toxin called tetanospasim that is excreted by the anaerobic bacterium, *Clostridium tetani*. Spores of *C. tetani* are found in soil and animal feces worldwide. The spores are hardy. They can survive up to 20 years and are resistant to heat and many disinfectants. Tetanus cannot be passed from person to person and becoming infected does not create prolonged natural immunity. Immunity can be achieved through vaccination, but even vaccine-produced immunity decreases over time. After receiving a complete series of childhood vaccinations, older children and adults need a tetanus booster in the form of Td or Tdap every 10 years.

C. tetani spores enter the body through a break in the skin that can be as minor as a paper cut or the prick of a thorn. Once in the body, they are activated and produce bacteria. In about one week, symptoms appear that include painful muscle contractions, muscle stiffness, difficulty swallowing, and heavy sweating. Between one-half and three-quarters of people with tetanus cannot open their jaw, thus the common name of lockjaw. About 1 in 10 people die.

Tetanus is uncommon in countries with comprehensive immunization programs. Fewer than 30 cases occur in the United States each year, all in unvaccinated or incompletely vaccinated individuals. People who inject illicit drugs are at highest risk because the materials used to dilute the drugs are sometimes contaminated with tetanus spores. In developing countries, the rate of tetanus is highest in newborns who acquire the disease through contaminated equipment used to cut the umbilical cord.

Pertussis

Pertussis is a respiratory infection commonly called whooping cough. It is caused by the bacterium *Bordetella pertussis* and is transmitted by face-to-face contact, sharing a confined space with an infected person, and contact with nasal and respiratory secretions of an infected person. Before 1992, pertussis vaccine was made using whole killed bacteria and the combination vaccine was called DPT. Whole killed pertussis bacteria caused most of the adverse reactions to the vaccine. To reduce adverse effects, an acellular version of pertussis vaccine was developed. Acellular pertussis uses only selected proteins that stimulate antibody production. By eliminating proteins that do not play a role in developing immunity, acellular pertussis causes fewer adverse effects.

Pertussis begins with symptoms similar to the common cold, but soon violent coughing develops that can last several minutes and makes breathing difficult. The "whoop" of whooping cough is the sound the person makes trying to breathe. Chronic coughing lasts six weeks or longer.

Worldwide, an estimated 48.5 million cases of pertussis and 295,000 deaths occur annually. In the United States, outbreaks occur every two to five years. In 2012, 48,277 cases and 20 deaths were reported to the CDC. In the past, most deaths occurred among infants too young to be vaccinated and in unvaccinated young children. However, 11- and 12-year-olds were hardest hit in the 2012 outbreak, suggesting that acellular pertussis vaccine might not provide extended immunity equivalent to the discontinued whole-cell vaccine. Children older than 12 years would have received the earlier whole-cell vaccine, while vaccinated younger children would still have immunity from the early childhood series of DTaP, leaving 11- and 12-year-olds vulnerable.

Administration of DTaP and DT Vaccines

DTaP is a combination vaccine given by intramuscular injection. DT lacks the pertussis component and can be given in situations where the individual cannot tolerate any pertussis vaccine. DTaP can be administered to children ages of six weeks through six years. The recommended schedule calls for five doses given at ages two, four, and six months, between fifteen and eighteen months, and between four and six years.

Administration of Tdap and Td

Tdap and Td are vaccines for children over age seven years and adults. A single dose of Tdap is recommended for children ages 11 (the preferred time) through 18 years, especially if these children have close contact with an infant too young to be vaccinated. Adults who have not received Tdap, which was licensed in the United States in 2005, should receive one dose of the vaccine. Otherwise, they should receive a Td booster every 10 years.

Pregnant women are given a single dose of Tdap between weeks 27 and 36 of each pregnancy. The antibodies the mother makes to the vaccine cross the placenta and provide some protection to the baby during the first weeks of life when its immune system is too immature for DTaP vaccination to be effective.

Adverse Effects

Adverse effects with DTaP usually are mild but quite common. One in four children develops redness, soreness, swelling at the injection site, and/or fever. These adverse effects are more common after the fourth or fifth dose. Mild effects include fussiness in about one-third of children, poor appetite (10 percent), and vomiting (2 percent). In about 3.3 percent of children, swelling may extend along the entire arm or leg for up to one week after the fourth or fifth injection.

Moderate adverse effects are less common and include seizures (twitching, jerking, or staring), which occur in about 1 of every 14,000 children, nonstop crying for three or more hours (one of every 1,000 children), and fever over 105°F (40.5°C) in 1 of every 16,000 children.

Severe adverse effects are rare. Serious allergic reactions occur less than once in one million doses. Long-term seizures, coma, and brain damage have been reported, but these conditions occur so infrequently that it is not clear if they result from exposure to the vaccine or from other causes.

Special Populations

DTaP should not be given, or should be given with special care, in certain situations. Parents should discuss any conditions that may alter the administration of the vaccine with their child's pediatrician.

- Children who have had a severe allergic reaction to a dose of DTaP should not complete the immunization series.
- Children who have experienced a brain or nervous system disease within seven days of vaccination with DTaP should not complete the immunization series.
- Moderately or severely ill children and adults should wait until they are healthy to be vaccinated.
- Parents of children who have had any of the moderate adverse effects listed above after vaccination should discuss the advisability of continuing immunization with DTaP with their pediatrician.

Postexposure Prophylaxis

Postexposure prophylaxis is the administration of a drug or vaccine after known or suspected exposure to a disease with the goal of preventing the disease or reducing its severity. Tdap may be given to any individuals exposed to a documented case of pertussis regardless of their current immunization status.

Individuals with a wound that may have exposed them to tetanus (e.g., a puncture wound, animal bite, or a wound contaminated with soil) are routinely given Td if their immunization status is unknown or if they have not had a Td booster dose within 10 years. ACIP also recommends that individuals injured in bombings or natural disasters where they are likely to have soil in their wounds receive a Td booster if their immunization status is unknown or if they have not had a Td booster within five years. Even in people who have had a recent booster shot, an additional one causes no increased health risks.

What Makes This Vaccine Controversial?

DTaP is less controversial than its predecessor DTwP, more commonly called DPT. DPT is the vaccine that gave life to the modern anti-vaccination movement in the United States and led to the formation anti-vaccination pressure groups. Parents claimed on anecdotal evidence that DPT caused autism and developmental delays. This controversy is discussed in Chapter 10. The newer DTaP formulation causes fewer adverse reactions. However, vaccine skeptics now object to this vaccine on the grounds that the vaccine is a combination vaccine, which they believe stresses their child's immune system. No single vaccine for every of component of DTaP is available.

Haemophilus Influenzae Type B

Haemophilus influenzae type b (Hib) is a bacterial disease. Despite the word *influenzae* in its name, it has no relationship to viral influenza. As many as three-quarters of adults have Hib bacteria in their nose and throat. They do not show symptoms, but they can spread the disease to children through face-to-face contact and respiratory droplets.

So long as Hib bacteria are confined to the nose and throat, they cause few problems. However, Hib can become invasive and enter other parts of the body, causing serious or fatal illness. Before a vaccine was available, invasive Hib was the leading cause of bacterial meningitis in children. Meningitis can leave children blind, deaf, paralyzed, or with brain damage. Symptoms include fever, drowsiness, and stiff neck. Hib can also cause pneumonia, bloodstream infections (bacteremia), and epiglottitis. Other pathogens besides Hib also cause these diseases.

Children under five years old are most at risk for Hib infection, with infants under one year most likely to experience permanent damage from the disease. Before an effective Hib vaccine came into widespread use in the early 1990s, there were between 20,000 and 25,000 serious cases of invasive Hib in the United States in children under age five each year. By 2012, only 25 cases were reported in this age group.

Administration of Hib Vaccine

Hib vaccine is a conjugate vaccine. Hib bacteria are encased in a polysaccharide coat. The immune system, especially in children less than two years old, does not respond strongly to vaccine that contains only polysaccharide from the bacterium. To solve this problem, vaccine makers create a conjugate vaccine by attaching a harmless protein to the polysaccharide coat. Immune system cells, even in infants, respond strongly enough to the protein–polysaccharide combination to create immunity.

Hib vaccines are intended for use in children between the ages of six weeks and five years. They are administered by intramuscular injection. Three Hib vaccines (PedvaxHIB, ActHIB, and Hiberix) are used in the United States. Their main difference is the type of protein added to the Hib polysaccharide, but they also have different administration schedules. Hib is also included in a two-vaccine combination for Hib and hepatitis B (Comvax) and a five-combination vaccine that immunizes against diphtheria, tetanus, pertussis, poliomyelitis, and Hib (Pentacel).

Hib vaccines that require four doses (ActHIB, Hiberix, MenHibRix, Pentacel) are recommended to be given at ages two, four, and six months with a fourth booster dose at twelve to fifteen months. Hib vaccines that require three doses (PedvaxHIB, Comvax) are given at two and four months with a booster at twelve to fifteen months. If the recommended sequence is interrupted, catch-up doses can be given without starting the series over. After age five, children are vaccinated against Hib only under special circumstances (see Special Populations later in the chapter).

Adverse Effects

Hib vaccine has some of the fewest adverse effects of any childhood vaccine. Those that it does have tend to be mild and transient, lasting only two or three days. These include redness and swelling at the injection site and a low fever. Serious allergic reaction is estimated to occur fewer than once in one million doses.

Special Populations

Children over age five years normally are not given Hib vaccine. Nevertheless, certain situations may change its recommended administration

schedule. Parents should discuss any conditions that may alter the administration of the vaccine with their child's pediatrician.

- Children under age six weeks should not receive Hib vaccine.
- Children who have had a severe allergic reaction to Hib vaccine
  (extremely rare) should not complete the immunization series.
- Moderately or severely ill children should not be vaccinated until
  they are healthy.
- Children ages one to five years with certain medical conditions are at
  higher risk of developing invasive Hib disease than healthy children
  and may need an altered administration schedule and/or an additional
  dose of vaccine. These include children receiving chemotherapy or
  radiation therapy, children with certain spleen abnormalities, and
  children with sickle cell disease or HIV infection.
- A supplemental dose of Hib vaccine is recommended two weeks before
  surgery for children undergoing nonemergency removal of the spleen.
- Unimmunized children ages five through eighteen years with HIV
  infection should receive one dose of the vaccine.
- All people older than five years who receive hematopoietic (blood
  cell producing) stem cell transplants should be revaccinated.

What Makes This Vaccine Controversial?

Hib is one of the least controversial childhood vaccines because of its
low rate of adverse reactions. The vaccine was introduced less than 25 years
ago, so many parents are familiar with Hib infection from their own childhood and are aware of its severity (a mortality rate of 5–10 percent and permanent deficits among 15–30 percent of survivors). This familiarity may
make them more willing to vaccinate their children against Hib.

Hepatitis A

Hepatitis A causes acute liver inflammation. It is found in the feces of
infected people and is transmitted by the fecal–oral route, most often by
contaminated food (especially raw shellfish and other uncooked foods),
contaminated water (usually from sewage spills), and poor hygiene. The
largest volume of virus is shed in feces one to two weeks before symptoms
occur. Once jaundice (yellowing of the skin due to liver damage) develops
at about two weeks, the amount of virus shed decreases substantially.

Symptoms are nonspecific and age-dependent. Many children younger
than age six years show no symptoms. A few have stomach pain and diarrhea. Older children and adults are likely to develop a fever, jaundice, dark

urine, abdominal pain, nausea, and fatigue. Symptoms can last up to two months with relapses within six months. There is no treatment, but the disease is rarely fatal.

Hepatitis A is uncommon in the United States. Only 2,007 cases were reported in 2016, a decrease of more than 90 percent since vaccination began. However, in 2018, an outbreak in Utah infected more than 4,000 people. Hepatitis A is common in countries where sanitation and water treatment are poor, including Mexico, parts of the Caribbean, Central America, South America, Asia (except Japan), Africa, the Middle East, and Eastern Europe. Since many young children in these areas acquire hepatitis A but show no symptoms, the worldwide prevalence of the disease is difficult to determine.

Although hepatitis A and hepatitis B sound similar, hepatitis A is an acute, or short-lived, disease. Once recovered, there normally is no permanent damage. Hepatitis B is a chronic disease that causes long-term serious liver damage that can lead to cirrhosis, liver cancer, and death. People need to receive separate vaccines to immunize against hepatitis A and hepatitis B. A combination vaccine against both diseases (Twinrix) is available only for adults.

Administration of Hepatitis A Vaccine

Hepatitis A vaccine is made of inactivated whole virus administered as an intramuscular injection. The *picornavirus* that causes hepatitis A was first isolated in 1973, and the first vaccine became available in the United States in 1995. The CDC recommended routine childhood vaccination beginning in 2006. Two different vaccines are used in the United States, Havrix and Vaqta. Both come in two formulations, one for children ages 12 months through 18 years and the other for adults age 19 years and older. Two doses of either vaccine create almost 100 percent immunity in both children and adults.

The CDC recommends that children receive the first dose between 12 and 23 months of age with a booster dose at least 6 months later. Children not vaccinated at this time can be given two catch-up doses later. Adults can begin the two-dose series at any time but should receive at least one dose one month before traveling to an area where hepatitis A is common.

Some groups are at higher risk of acquiring hepatitis A and should be routinely vaccinated. These include:

- Individuals of all ages traveling to areas where hepatitis A is common. At least one dose should be given at least 30 days before travel begins. For the best protection, the two-dose regimen should be completed before traveling.

- Members of a family planning to adopt or care for a child from an area where hepatitis A is common.
- Aid workers traveling to sites of natural disasters where water and sewage treatment is likely to be disrupted.
- Individuals with blood-clotting disorders.
- Men who have sex with men.
- Individuals who use street drugs.

Adverse Effects

Most people experience no or mild adverse effects from hepatitis A vaccination. Mild adverse effects include soreness at the injection site, headache, loss of appetite, and tiredness. Allergic reaction to the vaccine is serious but extremely rare.

Special Populations

Certain medical situations may change the recommended administration of hepatitis A vaccine. Individuals should discuss any conditions that may alter the use of the vaccine with their physician.

- Anyone who has had a severe allergic reaction to the antibiotic neomycin or to any other component of the vaccine should not be vaccinated.
- Moderately or severely ill individuals should wait until they are healthy to be vaccinated unless there is a pressing need.
- People with chronic liver conditions usually can be safely vaccinated.
- Sewer workers and plumbers may wish to consider vaccination because of their potential contact with fecal waste, although no outbreaks from this source have been recently reported in the United States.
- Food handlers may need to be vaccinated based on local occurrence of hepatitis A. Although food-related outbreaks are rare in the United States, an infected food handler was suspected of spreading the disease in the 2018 Utah outbreak.

What Makes This Vaccine Controversial?

Hepatitis A vaccine is not highly controversial, although many parents feel it is unnecessary and choose to have their children skip it.

Vaccination is strongly advised for individuals traveling to areas where the disease is common.

Hepatitis B

Hepatitis B is a liver disease caused by hepatitis B virus (HBV). The virus is transmitted by contact with body fluids from an infected person. Contact can occur through sexual activity; sharing needles, syringes, razors, or toothbrushes; unintended needle sticks or other accidental blood contact; and exposure to fluids from an infected mother as infant passes through the birth canal. HBV is 100 times more contagious than human immunodeficiency virus (HIV). One milliliter (one-fifth of a teaspoon) of infected blood is enough to pass the disease to a noninfected person. The virus can survive outside the body and cause infection for at least seven days.

Some infected individuals develop acute (short-term) hepatitis B infection, a brief illness that causes symptoms such as fatigue, loss of appetite, vomiting, and diarrhea about three months after exposure to the virus. Sometimes, especially in infants and children, acute infection progresses to chronic (long-term) hepatitis B infection. People with chronic HBV infection often show few symptoms and may not be aware that they are infected until the disease causes liver damage (cirrhosis) or liver cancer. An estimated 800,000 to 2.2 million Americans have chronic hepatitis B infection, and between 4,000 and 5,000 die of complications each year. Worldwide, the WHO estimates that 240 million people have chronic infection that causes 786,000 deaths annually.

The rate of hepatitis B in the United States has dropped by 82 percent since routine infant vaccination began in 1991, and the disease has practically been eliminated in native-born Americans under age 20. New infections occur most often in men between the ages of 25 and 44 years, usually through sexual activity or intravenous drug abuse.

Administration of Hepatitis B Vaccine

Hepatitis B vaccines are recombinant subunit vaccines. They cannot cause the disease they are intended to prevent. Three doses of hepatitis B vaccine produce complete immunity in 90 percent of people under 40 years old; coverage gradually decreases in people over age 40. The CDC recommends that newborns be vaccinated before being discharged from the hospital and ideally within 24 hours after birth. A second dose of vaccine is given at one month and the third at six months. The CDC recommends that babies not born in health care settings be vaccinated as soon as possible after birth.

One of two forms of the vaccine (Engerix-B and Recombivax HB) is normally given at birth because 90 percent of infected newborns go on to develop chronic hepatitis B. Two combination vaccines also contain the hepatitis B antigen. The combination vaccine Pediarix immunizes against hepatitis B, diphtheria, tetanus, pertussis, and polio. It can be given only between the ages of six weeks and seven years. Twinrix is a combination vaccine against hepatitis A and hepatitis B used to immunize at-risk adults. Among adults, health care workers and first responders are at especially high risk of contracting infection through accidental contact with contaminated blood.

If the timing of the recommended hepatitis B immunization schedule is interrupted, it is not necessary to start the series over again. The individual should simply follow the CDC catch-up schedule as soon as possible. Postexposure vaccination can reduce the risk of developing hepatitis B only if the individual is vaccinated very soon after exposure. Since symptoms of infection do not appear immediately, individuals often do not recognize that they have been exposed.

Adverse Effects

Hepatitis B vaccine causes few adverse effects. The most common are minor and transient. They include soreness at the injection site, fatigue, low-grade fever, headache, and dizziness. The most serious adverse effect is anaphylaxis, a life-threatening allergic reaction that occurs after about 1 in every 600,000 doses of the vaccine. People who are allergic to yeast, which is used in the manufacture of the vaccine, or any of the vaccine's other components should not be vaccinated.

Special Populations

Certain medical situations may change the recommended administration of hepatitis B vaccine. Parents should discuss any conditions that may alter the use of the vaccine with their child's pediatrician.

- Infants weighing less than 4.4 lb. (2,000 g) born to hepatitis B negative mothers should not be vaccinated until one month or hospital discharge.
- Immunocompromised individuals, including those with HIV infection, may respond less strongly to hepatitis B vaccine. These individuals should have blood tests to check the level of antibodies they form in response to inoculation. Booster shots may be needed.

- Adults on hemodialysis should have their antibody levels checked annually. Booster shots may be needed.
- Pregnant and breastfeeding women should delay receiving hepatitis B vaccine unless there is an urgent need. The safety of the vaccine in these populations has not been well studied.
- Moderately or severely ill individuals should delay vaccination until they are healthy unless there is an urgent need.
- People whose immunization status is unknown can receive the full three-dose course of vaccine. Extra doses of hepatitis B vaccine do not increase health risks.

What Makes This Vaccine Controversial?

Most anti-vaccination parents object to inoculating a newborn against a disease they are unlikely to encounter until they are much older and become sexually active. They also express concern that the child's immature immune system will be stressed by the antigens in the vaccine (see Chapter 11). Vaccinating infants born to hepatitis B–infected mothers is not controversial because of a documented risk of infected newborns developing chronic infection.

Human Papillomavirus

Forty types of papillomavirus are known to infect the genital areas of both men and women and the lining of the cervix in women. Some types of human papillomavirus (HPV) can cause cervical, vaginal, anal, penile, or throat cancer and may be implicated in esophageal cancer. Other types cause genital warts. HPV is transmitted by vaginal, oral, or anal sexual contact with an infected person, making HPV infection the most common sexually transmitted infection (STI) worldwide. Newborns can also acquire the virus from an infected mother while passing through the birth canal.

The CDC estimates that 79 million Americans are infected with HPV, with somewhere between 6 million and 14 million new infections occurring each year. Most of the new infections are in people ages 15–24 years. For many people, HPV infection resolves on its own with no complications. Depending on the type of HPV, some people develop genital warts. Genital warts can be treated but not cured. Recurrent outbreaks are common.

In the United States, about 26,000 HPV-associated cancers are newly diagnosed each year. Ninety-nine percent of cervical cancers and 71 percent of penile cancers are associated with HPV infection. In 2018, the American Cancer Society estimated that 8,580 new cases of anal cancer and 1,160 deaths, 2,320 new cases of penile cancer and 380 deaths, and 13,240 new cases of cervical cancer and 4,170 deaths would occur in the United States that year. Worldwide, more than 500,000 new cases of cervical cancer are diagnosed each year, causing an estimated 266,000 deaths annually. There is no cure for HPV infection, but as of 2018, three different vaccines were available in the United States to immunize against up to 9 of the 40 types of HPV.

Administration of HPV Vaccine

All three HPV vaccines are subunit vaccines made with recombinant DNA technology. They cannot cause HPV infection or cause cancer. A quadrivalent vaccine, HPV4 (Gardasil), was approved in 2006. It immunizes against HPV types 16 and 18, which together cause 70 percent of cervical cancers, and types 6 and 11, which cause 90 percent of genital warts. The vaccine is approved for males and females 9–26 years of age. A bivalent vaccine, HPV2 (Cervarix), was approved in 2009. It immunizes against HPV types 16 and 18, the types most often associated with cervical cancer, and is appropriate for females ages 10–25 years. This vaccine is not approved for males of any age. In December 2014, a nine-valent vaccine, HPV9 (Gardasil-9), was licensed in the United States. It immunizes against HPV types 6, 11, 16, 18, 31, 33, 45, 52, and 58 and is approved for use in males and females ages 9–26 years.

The recommended age for the first dose of HPV vaccine is 11 or 12 years. The goal is to immunize children before they are sexually active because HPV is extremely widespread, is highly contagious, and often causes no noticeable symptoms. Many people do not realize they are infected and pass the infection to their partners. Although HPV vaccines prevent certain types of HPV infection, they have no effect on infections the individual has already acquired. This is another reason for vaccinating at a young age. Children who are not vaccinated at the recommended age can be vaccinated up to age 26 years.

Before 2016, three doses of HPV vaccine were recommended for all eligible individuals. In late 2016, the CDC changed this recommendation, because evidence showed that two doses of HPV given six months apart to children ages 11 to 14 years produced a response equivalent to three doses in individuals ages 16 to 26 years. The first HPV vaccine dose is recommended at age 11 or 12 years. A second dose is given either one or two months after the first dose. A third dose for individuals over age 14 years is given six months after the first dose. If the series is interrupted, it does not need to be started over. Individuals who have started the series with

HPV4 can complete it with HPV9, but if the full series was completed using HPV4, revaccination with HPV9 is not recommended.

Adverse Effects

HPV vaccine has only mild adverse effects. Most common are redness, pain, and swelling at the injection site. About 10 percent of people develop a slightly elevated temperature. Allergic reaction to the vaccine or other serious adverse events has not been reported.

Special Populations

Certain medical situations may change the recommended administration of HPV vaccine.

Individuals should discuss any conditions that may alter use of the vaccine with their physician.

- Anyone who has had a severe allergic reaction to yeast protein or any other component of the vaccine should not be vaccinated.
- Anyone who has a severe reaction to a dose of HPV vaccine (extremely rare) should not complete the series.
- Pregnant women should wait to be vaccinated until after the birth of the child.
- Moderately or severely ill individuals should delay vaccination until they are healthy.
- Immunocompromised individuals should check with their physician, but most, including those with HIV infection, can be safely vaccinated.

What Makes This Vaccine Controversial?

HPV vaccine is one of the more controversial vaccines for children. Some parents object to vaccinating children against an STI when they are not sexually active. They feel this may encourage early sexual activity and/or give children the incorrect belief that they are protected against other STIs. This controversy is discussed in Chapter 11.

Influenza

Influenza is a highly contagious disease spread through tiny respiratory droplets that are sneezed or coughed into the air by a person who is infected with flu virus. The virus can also spread through direct contact, such as by kissing or drinking from the same glass as an infected person. Influenza is a cool weather disease. The CDC estimates that between

10 and 20 percent of all people in the United States contract influenza between November and March each year.

People are infectious one day before symptoms appear. Symptoms include fever, chills, headache, body aches, sore throat, runny nose, and dry cough. After about four days, symptoms diminish, but people remain contagious until symptoms completely disappear. For most people, influenza is unpleasant but not life threatening. For some, it can be fatal. Children under age two years, the elderly, and people who are immuno-compromised or have a heart or lung disease are the most likely to die from influenza or its complications.

Influenza weakens the body, increasing the chance of developing an opportunistic infection such as *Streptococcus pneumoniae* or *Haemophilus influenzae* that cause pneumonia. Between 100,000 and 200,000 people, mostly the very young and the elderly, are hospitalized in the United States each year with influenza or its complications, and 20,000–36,000 of them die. The WHO estimates that worldwide there are 3–5 million cases of influenza each year causing 250,000–500,000 deaths.

There are three types of influenza viruses called A, B, and C. Influenza C causes only mild illness, usually in children. Influenza B makes people sicker than influenza C but usually accounts for only 20 percent of flu cases. Influenza A is responsible for serious illness and widespread epidemics. Influenza viruses mutate frequently, creating new strains that cause infection in humans. Other strains cause disease in chickens, ducks, wild birds, pigs, horses, ferrets, whales, and seals.

Vaccines against influenza are different from other vaccines because their composition must change every year to keep up with the mutating virus. Past immunizations and previous exposure to influenza do not provide protection against new strains. In 1952, the WHO established the Global Influenza Surveillance and Response System. As part of this program, laboratories worldwide test hundreds of thousands of samples from patients with influenza to determine which strains are most common and to detect the emergence of new strains. They use this information to give advice on which strains should be included in the vaccines for the following year. The prevalence of influenza in any year depends on how well the strains in the vaccine match the strains of influenza present in the community and how many people have been vaccinated.

Administration of Influenza Vaccine

Influenza vaccination is recommended for all people over age six months with the few exceptions noted below under Special Populations. Revaccination with the current formulation of vaccine is recommended well before the onset of cool weather. It takes two weeks to develop adequate antibodies to provide immunity, so people are encouraged to get vaccinated before flu appears in their community.

Each year, influenza vaccine protects only against either three A strains (trivalent vaccine) or three A and one B strain (quadrivalent vaccine), so it is still possible to contract the disease if the strains in the vaccine do not match the strains common in the community. Over the years, flu vaccine effectiveness has ranged from about 36 percent to 72 percent. The effective rate for the 2016–2017 influenza season was 43 percent. Early reports suggest the 2017–2018 vaccine was even less effective.

Multiple types of influenza vaccine are used in the United States. Not all vaccines are appropriate for all people. Inactivated influenza vaccines, the most common type of flu vaccine, are produced by growing the virus in chicken eggs, harvesting it, and then inactivating it with chemicals. All vaccines produced using chicken eggs contain a small amount of egg protein. The virus in cell culture–based inactivated vaccine (Flucelvax) is grown in canine kidney cells and then inactivated. Recombinant influenza vaccine (Flublok) is made in the laboratory using only proteins from the coat of influenza viruses and not the whole virus. These two vaccines do not contain egg protein and can be used to vaccinate individuals with egg allergy.

Adverse Effects

Common adverse effects of influenza vaccine in children and adults from all versions of the vaccine include soreness or redness at the injection site, runny nose, nasal congestion, cough, headache, and muscle ache. Mild fever is more common in children than in adults but is still infrequent. People who are allergic to eggs may experience an allergic reaction. To avoid this, they can receive Flucelvax or Flublok. Children who receive influenza vaccine at the same time as DTaP or pneumococcal vaccine (PCV13) may have an increased risk of febrile seizures.

Questions have been raised about whether vaccination against influenza increases the risk of developing Guillain-Barré syndrome (GBS), a rare neurological disorder. Studies have found that influenza vaccination does not increase the risk of GBS in people who have never had the disorder but that risk of recurrence, although rare, is slightly higher in people who have had GBS and recovered.

Special Populations

Although immunization against influenza is generally recommended for everyone above age six months, certain medical situations may dictate which type of vaccine is most appropriate. Only a very few individuals should not be vaccinated. Individuals should discuss any conditions that may alter administration of the vaccine with their physician.

- Anyone who has had a severe allergic reaction to a previous dose of influenza vaccine or any of its components should not be vaccinated. People who have egg allergy should tell their health care provider and usually can be vaccinated with a formulation that does not contain egg protein.
- Anyone who has developed GBS within six weeks of having received influenza vaccine should not be vaccinated. People who have had GBS and recovered should discuss the advisability of vaccination with their physician.
- Moderately or severely ill individuals should wait until they are healthy to be vaccinated.
- Children between the ages of six months and eight years receiving influenza vaccine for the first time should receive two doses at least 28 days apart.
- Caretakers and family members of people who are immunocompromised should not receive live attenuated vaccine. Live virus can be shed for up to three weeks and can transmit influenza to an immunocompromised person.
- Pregnant women can safely be vaccinated with any type of influenza vaccine except live attenuated vaccine during any trimester of pregnancy. Use of intranasally administered live attenuated vaccine was temporarily discontinued in 2016 but has been reinstated for use in the 2018–2019 influenza season.

What Makes This Vaccine Controversial?

The low rate of effectiveness coupled with the perception even among people who accept other vaccines that influenza is not a serious disease makes some people skeptical that the benefits of influenza vaccine outweigh the risks. Many childcare and health care facilities require their employees to get annual flu shots. Although courts have ruled that this is legal, anti-vaccinationists feel the requirement infringes on their right to make their own health care decisions (see Chapter 12).

Measles, Mumps, and Rubella

The vaccine that immunizes against measles, mumps, and rubella (MMR) is given as a single injection in the United States. Single-antigen vaccines against each individual disease are available in some countries but not in the United States. The combination vaccine, available since 1971, contains live attenuated viruses and provides long-term immunity to all three diseases. A combination vaccine against measles, mumps, rubella, and varicella (MMRV; brand name ProQuad) was licensed in 2005.

Measles

Measles, also called rubeola (not to be confused with rubella or German measles), is highly contagious. It spreads by respiratory droplets exhaled by an infected person. If 100 unvaccinated people are in a room with an infected person, on average 90 will develop measles. The virus can remain infective in a sheltered space such as a closed room for up to two hours. People are contagious four days before and four days after the measles rash appears.

Measles is characterized by a fever of 103–105°F (39.4–40.5°C), rash, conjunctivitis (pink eye), runny nose, cough, headache, and body aches. Symptoms last around two weeks. About one-third of people, especially those under age five years and adults, develop complications. Complications can be minor (e.g., ear infection), permanent, or fatal. Serious complications include pneumonia (the most common cause of measles-related death), encephalitis (brain inflammation), convulsions, deafness, blindness, and intellectual disabilities.

Before a measles vaccine was licensed in 1963, on average 500,000 cases of measles and 500 measles-related deaths were reported in the United States each year. About 90 percent of children contracted the disease by age 15 years. By 2000, native measles was declared eliminated in the United States. Nevertheless, travelers arriving from parts of the world where measles is active continue to bring the disease into the country.

Outbreaks occur in the United States every few years, primarily, but not exclusively, among people who have refused vaccination. In 2017, 79 measles cases were reported to the Minnesota Department of Health. This compares to a *total* of 56 cases reported in Minnesota during the previous 19 years. Only two of the children in this outbreak had been vaccinated. Europe also sees periodic outbreaks of measles due to low vaccination rates. Romania reported 7,491 cases of the disease and 31 deaths during the first 6 months of 2017. During the same period, Italy reported 3,346 measles cases and 2 deaths. Worldwide, 400 children die each day of measles or complications of the disease.

Mumps

Mumps is a viral infection spread by respiratory droplets and direct contact. The virus reproduces in the nose, throat, and surrounding lymph glands for 12–25 days, after which it spreads to other tissues and can cause swelling and inflammation in the salivary glands, meninges, pancreas, kidney, ovaries, or testes. Swelling of the salivary (parotid) glands located under the ear and along the jaw on one of both sides is the most prominent sign. Before swelling occurs, symptoms of mumps are nonspecific—body aches, fatigue, and low fever.

Complications from mumps include orchitis (testicular swelling) in some men past puberty, most often only on one side. Rarely do mumps cause male sterility. Other complications are uncommon. Swelling occurs in the ovaries of about 7 percent of postpuberty women but does not affect their fertility. Other complications include aseptic meningitis (a condition in which inflammation of the membranes covering is not caused by a pathogen), deafness, or hearing loss (transient or permanent).

As with measles, most mumps cases in the United States originate from people arriving from countries where mumps is common. Fewer than 60 percent of countries who belong to the WHO routinely administer mumps vaccine, putting unvaccinated visitors to those countries at high risk for contracting the disease. The CDC reported 6,353 cases of mumps in 2016, including an outbreak that affected 40 people at Harvard University.

Rubella

Rubella is a mild viral infection spread by respiratory droplets. Symptoms include low fever, light rash that begins on the face and spreads downward, and swollen glands. As many as half of all people who contract rubella show no diagnostic symptoms. Complications are rare in healthy children. A large percentage of adult women develop joint pain and stiffness that can last up to one month.

The most serious outcomes of rubella infection appear in the developing fetus of a woman who contracts the disease during pregnancy. The virus that causes rubella can cross the placenta and cause birth defects, a condition called congenital rubella syndrome. The most serious consequences occur when the woman is infected during the first trimester of pregnancy. Eighty-five percent of babies born to mothers infected during this time have birth defects. Rubella-caused defects are rare if the infection is acquired after the twentieth week of pregnancy. Congenital rubella syndrome can lead to the following complications in the fetus: death, miscarriage, or preterm delivery; deafness (most common defect); eye defects such as cataracts, glaucoma, and retinopathy; heart defects; spleen and liver damage; seizures; and intellectual and developmental delays.

Routine vaccination has made rubella rare in the United States today. An estimated 91 percent of all Americans are immune to the disease. Rubella is still common in parts of the Russian Federation, Europe, and many developing countries, putting unvaccinated travelers at risk.

Administration of MMR Vaccine

Both MMR and MMRV (the V stands for varicella, the chickenpox vaccine) are given as subcutaneous (under the skin but not in the muscle) injections. Two doses are recommended. The first should occur between the first birthday and 15 months. Any dose given before the first birthday must be repeated after the child reaches one year. The second dose can be given as early as 28 days after the first dose but is routinely given between ages four and six years, ideally before the child starts school. As of April 2018, a recommendation for a third dose of MMR during times of disease outbreak was under consideration.

The CDC recommends that to decrease the chance of febrile seizures, children receiving the first dose of MMR be given a separate dose of varicella vaccine rather than the combined MMRV vaccine, even when the vaccines are given at the same office visit. MMRV, if desired, can be used for the second dose up to age 13 years. MMR can be given to all children over one year and to adults. Two doses of MMR provide 99 percent coverage against measles, 88 percent coverage against mumps, and 95 percent coverage against rubella.

Adults born after 1957 who do not have documented proof of vaccination should receive a single dose of MMR. The exception is pregnant women. Women who wish to become pregnant must wait at least 28 days after vaccination before trying to conceive. Should an adult be deficient in immunity to one of the diseases in the vaccine—for example, if a man had measles and rubella as a child but never contracted mumps—it is safe to vaccinate with MMR. The extra dose of MMR vaccine against diseases to which an individual is already immune causes no health problems.

Adverse Effects

Allergic reactions can occur but are rare with MMR vaccine. Fever is the most common side effect. It is associated with the measles component of the vaccine. Five to fifteen percent of people who develop a fever have a temperature of 103°F (39.4°C) or higher 5–12 days after vaccination. The fever lasts one to two days and febrile seizures are possible, especially in children. Children ages 12–23 months who receive MMRV instead of MMR as a first dose are more likely to develop a high fever.

Other adverse effects of MMR vaccination include joint pain (associated with the rubella component), soreness at the injection site, and mild rash (associated with the mumps component). Low blood platelet count (thrombocytopenia) occurs two to three weeks after vaccination in 1 of every 30,000–40,000 people and can be serious.

Special Populations

Certain medical situations may change the recommended administration of MMR and MMRV. Parents should discuss any conditions that may alter the administration of the vaccine with their child's pediatrician.

- Infants traveling internationally can receive a dose of MMR vaccine as early as six months but must be revaccinated with two additional doses after their first birthday.
- Anyone who has had a severe allergic reaction to the antibiotic neomycin or any other component of the vaccine should not be vaccinated.
- Pregnant women or those trying to become pregnant should wait to be vaccinated until after the birth of the child.
- Immunocompromised individuals with leukemia, lymphoma, generalized malignancy, or immune deficiency diseases should not be vaccinated.
- Individuals who have a suppressed immune system from taking steroid drugs or chemotherapy should wait one month (steroids) or three months (chemotherapy) after treatment has stopped before being vaccinated.
- People with a family history of seizures should not be vaccinated.
- People who have recently received a blood product should wait to be vaccinated.
- Moderately or severely ill individuals should delay vaccination until they are healthy.
- Children allergic to eggs can be safely vaccinated.

What Makes This Vaccine Controversial?

MMR vaccine is the source of the most widespread misinformation and controversy over vaccine safety. Anti-vaccinationists have linked the measles component of the vaccine to autism spectrum disorder (ASD) and developmental delays despite multiple studies finding no link between them. As of 2018, the Institute of Medicine and the American Academy of Pediatrics had independently reviewed the evidence regarding this potential link. Both groups have concluded that evidence does not support any association between MMR vaccine and ASD. This controversy is discussed in Chapter 10.

Meningococcal Vaccines

Meningococcal disease is caused by the bacterium *Neisseria meningitidis*. Six strains of this bacterium (A, B, C, W, Y, and X) can cause meningitis, bloodstream infection, and sometimes pneumonia or arthritis. These diseases also have other causes.

N. meningitidis lives in the throats of about 10 percent of healthy people without causing symptoms. Although these people are not sick, they can spread the disease through close contact such as kissing, sharing food and drinks, or being in the same room or house with someone for more than four hours a day. Risk of developing meningococcal disease is age related. Children under age one year and teens and young adults ages 16–23 years living in close contact with other young people (e.g., in college dorms, prisons, military barracks) are at highest risk. Individuals of any age who are immunocompromised are also at high risk of developing meningococcal disease.

Meningococcal disease spreads less easily than influenza or measles, but symptoms develop abruptly and intensely. These include sudden onset of high fever, headache, stiff neck, sensitivity to light, nausea, and vomiting that can rapidly progress to hypotension (low blood pressure), shock, coma, and death. A child can appear healthy and 12 hours later be near death.

Even with treatment, 10–20 percent of people with meningococcal disease die. The rate is highest (about 33 percent) for people who develop bloodstream infection. About 12 percent of survivors are left with permanent damage such as limb amputation, skin-grafting scars, hearing loss, kidney damage, seizures, and intellectual disabilities. Worldwide, an estimated 500,000 cases of meningococcal disease occur each year and at least 50,000 people die.

Administration of Meningococcal Vaccines

In 2017, two meningococcal vaccines, Menomune, a polysaccharide quadrivalent vaccine, and MenHibRix, a conjugate combination vaccine, were discontinued in the United States due to low demand. Two vaccines,

Table 5.1 Types of Meningococcal Vaccines

Type of Vaccine	Brand Names	Strains Covered
Conjugate quadrivalent (MCV4)	Menactra	A, C, W, Y
	Menveo	
Recombinant	Bexsero	B
	Trumenba	

Menactra and Menveo, exist that protect against four strains (A, C, W, and Y) that cause most human disease. Two other vaccines, Bexsero and Trumenba, protect against strain B. No vaccine exists against strain X. Consequently, no single vaccine protects against all five strains, and several different vaccines exist to meet the needs of different age groups. Table 5.1 shows the vaccines as of 2018 and the strains they protect against.

Meningococcal bacteria are encased in a polysaccharide coat. The immune system of children younger than two years does not create immunity in response to a vaccine that contains only polysaccharide from the bacterium. To solve this problem, vaccine makers attach a harmless protein to the polysaccharide material. The added protein stimulates adequate immune system response to protect against disease.

Conjugate meningococcal vaccines (MCV4) protect against strains A, C, W, and Y, but do not provide protection against strain B, a common cause of disease in the United States. The MCV4 vaccine Menveo is approved for people ages 2 months to 55 years and Menactra for ages 9 months to 55 years. They are administered by intramuscular injection. Although approved for use in children under age two, the CDC recommends these vaccines only for a select group of young children (see Special Populations for these vaccines), not for routine vaccination of all children. The dosage schedule for special population children varies by age.

The CDC recommends routine vaccination with a MCV4 vaccine for children ages 11–18 years. Ideally, preteens should receive one dose of the vaccine between ages 11 and 12 years with a booster at age 16. Because college-age individuals are at high risk for contracting meningococcal disease, some universities require proof of vaccination before a student may enroll.

Two separate vaccines (Bexsero and Trumenba) provide protection against only meningococcal strain B. Although they protect against the same strain, the series should be completed using a single brand of vaccine. Neither vaccine is approved for children under age 10 years. Bexsero is a recombinant vaccine for people ages 10–25 years. It is given as an intramuscular injection. Two doses are needed to confer immunity and should be given one month apart.

Trumenba is a recombinant vaccine also approved for people ages 10–25 years. It can be given intramuscularly on a two-dose schedule with six months between the first and second injection or on a three-dose schedule with one month between the first and second injection and a third injection six months after the first dose. The preferred schedule depends on the risk level to the individual for contracting meningococcal disease.

Adverse Effects

All meningococcal vaccines cause only mild adverse effects. The most common are pain and soreness at the injection site, headache, and fatigue. Allergic reaction to the vaccine is serious but extremely rare.

Special Populations

Certain medical situations may change the recommended administration of meningococcal vaccine. Individuals should discuss any conditions that may alter the use of the vaccine with their physician. Some individuals should not receive meningococcal vaccine or should delay vaccination.

- Anyone who has had a severe allergic reaction to any component of the vaccine should not be vaccinated.
- Unless there is an urgent need, pregnant or breastfeeding women should wait to be vaccinated until the birth of the child or until they are not breastfeeding, as these vaccines have not been well studied in this population.
- Moderately or severely ill individuals should wait to be vaccinated until they are healthy.

Some people should get the vaccine even when they are out of the recommended age range. These include

- children and adults who have no spleen, a damaged spleen, or sickle cell disease;
- children and adults who lack certain complement proteins necessary for immune function;
- children and adults traveling to sub-Saharan Africa between December and June when meningococcal disease is common;
- adults who work with *N. meningitidis* in the laboratory or in a manufacturing environment;

- members in a community where there is an outbreak of meningococcal disease and their risk of exposure is high;
- individuals taking the drug eculizumab (Soliris). Administering this vaccine to someone taking Soliris can cause fatal illness. The vaccine must be administered a minimum of two weeks before the first dose of Soliris;
- immunosuppressed and immunocompromised individuals who may not respond strongly to the vaccine and have reduced immunity.

What Makes These Vaccines Controversial?

The low rate of adverse effects caused by meningococcal vaccines and the fact that many of them are given to adults, who can ignore or refuse vaccination if they find the vaccine objectionable, make them minimally controversial.

Pneumococcal Vaccines

Pneumococcal vaccines immunize against pneumococcal disease caused by certain strains of the bacterium *Streptococcus pneumoniae,* also called pneumococcus. Pneumonia can be caused by other bacteria, viruses, and fungi, but pneumococcus is a leading cause of invasive, life-threatening pneumonia. Infection with pneumococcus can also cause bacteremia (bloodstream infection), meningitis, and empyema (accumulation of pus between the lung and chest wall), all of which can be fatal. The bacterium is also responsible for less severe diseases including some ear and sinus infections.

As of 2018, about 100 different strains of *S. pneumoniae* had been isolated. The bacterium lives in the nose and throat of about one-quarter of the population without causing symptoms. These people can spread pneumococcal disease through sneezing, coughing, and saliva. Often parents with no symptoms infect their infants. Pneumococcal disease is an opportunistic infection that often follows another respiratory infection, especially influenza.

Two pneumococcal vaccines are used in the United States. A pneumococcal conjugate vaccine known as PCV13 (Prevnar 13) is given to infants, some children, and adults. A second pneumococcal vaccine, PPSV23 (Pneumovax 23), is given only to adults.

PCV13 protects against 13 common strains of *S. pneumoniae* that are responsible for about 60 percent of all invasive cases of pneumococcal pneumonia in children. In the United States before routine vaccination, *S. pneumoniae* was responsible for about 13,000 cases of bacteremia, 700 cases of meningitis, and 200 deaths in children each year. Worldwide, pneumococcal pneumonia causes about 1.2 million deaths annually in children under age five years.

A polysaccharide pneumococcal vaccine, PPSV23 (Pneumovax 23), is given to adults and children over age two years with specific medical conditions. It protects against 23 common strains of pneumococcus that cause severe, invasive disease. In the United States, about 400,000 people are hospitalized every year with pneumococcal pneumonia, and 18,000 older adults die from the disease.

Administration of Pneumococcal Conjugate Vaccine PCV13

PCV13 is a conjugate vaccine licensed in 2010. It replaced an earlier conjugate vaccine, PCV7, which was first used in 2000. *S. pneumoniae* is encased in a polysaccharide coat. The immune system of children younger than two years does not respond strongly to vaccines containing only polysaccharide from the bacterium. To solve this problem, vaccine makers attach a harmless protein to the polysaccharide material to stimulate the immune system. Even infant immune systems respond strongly enough to the protein–polysaccharide combination to protect against pneumococcal disease.

The recommended childhood schedule for vaccination with PCV13 consists of doses at 2, 4, and 6 months with a booster shot at 12–15 months given as an intramuscular injection. The vaccine can be given at the same time as other vaccines such as DTaP that conform to this schedule. Children not vaccinated before seven months of age should follow a catch-up schedule. Healthy children between the ages of two and five years who have received no doses of PCV13 need only a single dose. PCV13 is also recommended for all adults over age 65 and younger adults with certain medical conditions (see Special Populations for this vaccine). The vaccine is given even if the individual has received PPSV23. Recommendations for PCV13 administration for adults will be reevaluated in 2018.

Adverse Effects of PCV13

Adverse effects of PCV13 tend to be common but mild and transient. About half of all children receiving the vaccine become drowsy, have diminished appetite, and develop tenderness and redness at the injection site. About one-third of children show swelling at the injection site and a mild fever. One-fifth of them have a fever higher than 102.2°F (39°C). Most babies become fussy and irritable. Adults report similar mild reactions along with chills, headache, and muscle ache.

Special Populations

PCV13 should not be given, should be given on a different schedule, or given to older children and adults in certain situations. Individuals should discuss any conditions that may alter the administration of the vaccine with their physician.

- Individuals who are allergic to any components of PCV13 should not be vaccinated.
- Children who receive PCV13 at the same time as inactivated influenza vaccine may have an increased risk of febrile seizures. Parents should discuss this possibility with their pediatrician.
- Moderately or severely ill children and adults should wait until they are healthy to be vaccinated.
- Children ages two to six years who are immunocompromised or have chronic heart or lung disease, diabetes, cerebral spinal fluid (CSF) leak, cochlear implant, sickle cell disease, or other blood diseases should be given two doses of PCV13 at least eight weeks apart.
- Adults over age 18 years who are immunocompromised, have had a splenectomy (spleen removal), or have sickle cell disease, HIV infection, leukemia, lymphoma, Hodgkin disease, multiple myeloma, generalized malignancy, chronic renal failure, cochlear implants, or CSF leak should receive a dose of PCV13 vaccine before receiving PPSV23. If an individual has already received a dose of PPSV23, a special timing schedule must be followed for vaccination with PCV13 and future doses of PPSV23.

Administration of Polysaccharide Vaccine PPSV23

PPSV23 contains polysaccharide from the outer coating of 23 strains of *S. pneumonia*. The vaccine has been in use since 1983 and replaces a vaccine against 14 strains that is no longer manufactured. PPSV23 is ineffective in children under age two years. PPSV23 is between 60 percent and 70 percent effective in preventing invasive pneumococcal disease caused by the 23 strains included in the vaccine.

PPSV23 is recommended for all adults ages 65 years and older, even if they have received PCV13. The vaccine is also recommended for immunocompromised individuals over age two years and adults younger than age 65 years with specific medical conditions (see Special Populations for this vaccine). Revaccination for healthy people is recommended five years after the initial shot for people over age 65, as immunity decreases over time, especially in the elderly. Specific time intervals must elapse between the administration of PPSV23 and PCV13.

Adverse Effects of PPSV23

Between one-third and one-half of people vaccinated with PPSV23 report pain, redness, and some swelling at the injection site. These adverse effects are transient, usually lasting less than two days, and are more common after the second dose than after the first. Fever and muscle pain are uncommon (less than 1 percent of people), and serious adverse effects are rare.

Special Populations

Certain medical situations may change the recommended administration of PPSV23. Individuals should discuss any conditions that may alter use of the vaccine or timing of vaccination with their physician.

- People who have a severe allergy to any of the components of the vaccine should not be vaccinated.
- Moderately or severely ill individuals should delay vaccination until they are healthy.
- Immunocompromised people over age two years, including those who have had a splenectomy or have sickle cell disease, HIV infection, leukemia, lymphoma, Hodgkin disease, multiple myeloma, or chronic renal failure, should receive PPSV23 before age 65, but should not receive a second dose until after they reach age 65, even if that period is longer than the recommended five-year interval between doses.
- Adults age 19 and older who have asthma or smoke cigarettes should be vaccinated before age 65 years.
- In certain Native American populations at high risk for pneumococcal pneumonia, people over age two years should be vaccinated:
- Specific time intervals must be observed in administering PPSV23 to individuals who have already been vaccinated with PCV13 and vice versa. Individuals should alert their physician if they have previously received either of these vaccines.
- Individuals whose vaccination status is unknown or unclear can be vaccinated.

What Makes These Vaccines Controversial?

Pneumococcal vaccines are rarely controversial. Most criticism of them comes from the fact that they do not protect against all strains of pneumococcal bacteria. People may believe the vaccine has failed if they become sick from a strain not included in the vaccine. In addition, because of an aging immune system, vaccination of older adults is not as effective as vaccination of children.

Polio Vaccine–Inactivated

Poliomyelitis is a contagious viral disease with variable effects ranging from few to no symptoms (about 72 percent of people) to headaches, fever, stomach pain, and vomiting (about 25 percent) to permanent paralysis and death (less than 1 percent). The virus lives in the gastrointestinal tract and is spread by contact with contaminated stool (fecal–oral route) and by airborne droplets from infected individuals.

In the first half of the 20th century, polio paralyzed on average 10,000 children annually in the United States. An epidemic in the early 1950s killed about 6,000 people and paralyzed 27,000 more. With the development of a polio vaccine, native disease was eliminated in the United States in 1979. Thanks to the work of the Global Alliance for Vaccines and Immunization and the Global Polio Eradication Initiative, both international public–private partnerships, in the first half of 2018, Afghanistan reported only 10 cases of wild polio and Pakistan 3 cases. Two polio vaccines, oral polio vaccine (OPV) and inactivated polio vaccine (IPV) are in use worldwide. Only IPV is used in the United States. (See Vaccines Not Used in the United States for information on OPV.)

Administration of Inactivated Polio Vaccine

IPV uses inactivated whole virus to stimulate antibody production. Because the virus is incapable of reproducing, it cannot cause polio. The vaccine is given as an intramuscular injection in the thigh of young children and the arm of older children. The recommended schedule for IPV administration calls for four doses, the first two given at 2 and 4 months, a third dose between 6 and 18 months, and a booster dose between the ages of 4 and 6 years.

IPV is included in several combination vaccines such as the four-vaccine combination that immunizes against diphtheria, tetanus, pertussis, and polio; the five-vaccine combination against hepatitis b, diphtheria, tetanus, pertussis, and polio; and the five-combination vaccine against diphtheria, tetanus, pertussis, poliomyelitis, and Hib. Combination vaccines have administration schedules and age restrictions that differ from IPV. In meeting these schedules, children given a combination vaccine may receive a fifth dose of IPV. This causes no health complications. Ninety percent of children are immune to polio after two doses of IPV and 99 percent after three doses, but the duration of immunity is uncertain.

Adverse Effects

IPV causes few adverse effects, the most common being temporary soreness at the injection site. The vaccine contains small amounts of the antibiotics streptomycin, polymyxin B, and neomycin. People allergic to these antibiotics could have a severe allergic reaction to IPV.

Adverse effects of combination vaccines are the same as for each individual vaccine.

Special Populations

Certain medical situations may change the recommended administration of IPV. Parents should discuss any conditions that may alter the administration of the vaccine with their child's pediatrician.

- Individuals with a severe allergy to any of the components of IPV, including the antibiotics neomycin, streptomycin, or polymyxin B, should not be vaccinated.
- Anyone who has had a severe reaction to a dose IPV should not complete the immunization series.
- Moderately or severely ill individuals should delay vaccination until they are healthy unless there is an urgent need.
- Adults normally do not receive IPV, but adults such as humanitarian aid workers and military members traveling to areas where polio is active and people who work with *poliovirus* in the laboratory or in vaccine manufacturing settings should consider receiving a booster shot of IPV. Adults who have never been vaccinated should receive a three-dose series.

What Makes This Vaccine Controversial?

Many anti-vaccinationists in developed countries believe vaccination against polio is unnecessary since the disease has been eliminated in most countries including the entire Western Hemisphere, where the last case was recorded in 1993 (see Chapter 11). As of 2018, polio was reported in only a few places in the world. Nevertheless, war, political hostility to vaccination, and natural disasters still create openings for its resurgence. Vaccination is recommended until the disease is eradicated worldwide. Eradication is possible because, like smallpox and measles, only humans contract polio; there is no animal reservoir for the disease.

Rotavirus

Rotavirus is a virus that infects the lining of the intestine and causes high fever, vomiting, and severe diarrhea. There are multiple strains. Rotavirus is especially dangerous to infants because loss of large amounts of fluid can quickly cause fatal dehydration. Before a rotavirus vaccine became available, almost every child under age five years contracted the disease. The virus caused between 2.1 and 3.2 million cases of diarrhea in the United States each year, resulting in about 250,000 emergency room visits, as many as 70,000 hospitalizations, and up to 60 deaths. Since 2006, the vaccine has prevented 74–87 percent of all rotavirus illnesses in the United States, and severe cases of rotavirus-caused diarrhea have decreased between 85 percent and 98 percent.

Worldwide, rotavirus is the leading cause of dehydration in children. It causes about 125 million cases of diarrhea and between 500,000 and 527,000 deaths each year. The problem is especially acute in developing countries where access to clean water, rehydration fluids, and medical care are often limited. In poor and developing countries, 80 percent of infants contract the disease during their first year of life when they are most vulnerable.

Administration of Rotavirus Vaccine

Rotavirus vaccines are given only to infants. Two rotavirus vaccines are available in the United States as of 2018; additional vaccines are used in other countries. Rotarix is a live attenuated vaccine that protects against one strain of rotavirus. RotaTeq is a recombinant subunit vaccine that protects against five strains of rotavirus.

Rotavirus vaccines are given orally, beginning no earlier than six weeks of age. Rotarix requires a two-dose regimen. The recommended schedule is to give the first dose at two months and the second at four months. The first dose should not be given after age 14 weeks and 6 days, and the last dose should be given before the baby reaches 24 weeks of age.

RotaTeq is given in a three-dose series at two, four, and six months. The first dose should not be given after age 14 weeks and 6 days, and the last dose should be given before the baby reaches 32 weeks of age. Children who have not received three doses by the age of 32 weeks do not receive catch-up doses, as the effects of rotavirus are less lethal in older children.

Adverse Effects

Most babies experience no adverse effects from rotavirus vaccine. For those who do, the most common are fussiness or irritability, mild diarrhea, vomiting, and runny nose. Very rarely babies who have recently been vaccinated develop a type of bowel blockage called intussusception in which one part of the intestine slides into and blocks an adjacent part. This condition also occurs in unvaccinated babies for unknown reasons. Intussusception is a medical emergency requiring surgery. Studies have found that immunization against rotavirus increases the likelihood of intussusception over the naturally occurring or background rate by an amount estimated at between 1 in 20,000–100,000 infants.

Special Populations

Rotavirus vaccine should not be given or should be given with special care in certain situations. Parents should discuss any conditions that may alter the administration of the vaccine with their child's pediatrician.

- Babies who have had intussusception or another bowel blockage should not receive rotavirus vaccine.
- Babies born with severe combined immunodeficiency should not be vaccinated.
- Babies who have a severe allergic reaction to a dose of rotavirus vaccine should not complete the immunization series.
- Moderately or severely ill babies should not be vaccinated until they are healthy.
- Parents of babies born with gastrointestinal abnormalities should consult their physician about their child's risks.
- Parents of babies with weakened immune systems, such as those with HIV infection, taking steroid drugs, or who are receiving cancer treatment, should consult their physician about benefits and risks of vaccination.
- Babies can shed live rotavirus in their stool. If a family member is immunocompromised, the risk to this individual of contracting rotavirus diarrhea should be considered against the benefit to the baby.

What Makes This Vaccine Controversial?

Some vaccine-skeptic parents consider rotavirus a disease of poor, underdeveloped countries. They point out that many of the babies who die in developing countries do so because of lack of access to health care. Since good health care is readily accessible in the United States and other developed countries, these parents consider the vaccine unnecessary. This is discussed in Chapter 11.

Shingles

Shingles, also called herpes zoster, is caused by a reactivation of *varicella zoster,* the same virus that causes chickenpox. Chickenpox symptoms disappear within about two weeks. However, the *varicella zoster* virus enters nerve cells where it remains inactive, often for as many as 30–40 years. If the virus is reactivated, the individual develops shingles. The mechanism for reactivation is not well understood, but it appears to be connected to weakening of the immune system. Most shingles develop in people over age 60 years, although the virus can reactivate in much younger people who are immunocompromised (e.g., HIV infected; receiving chemotherapy).

Shingles is a painful but not life-threatening disease. The first sign is itching, burning, or a painful sensation on the skin. This is followed in one to five days by a rash that usually develops only on one side of the body. The rash is accompanied by pain and often headache and low fever. The rash evolves into fluid-filled blisters that crust over in about two weeks.

About 20 percent of people who develop shingles experience long-lasting pain called postherpetic neuralgia (PHN) so severe that it interferes with activities such as bathing, dressing, and sleeping. Pain usually is in the area where the rash was present and can last for months after the rash disappears. As of 2018, there was no treatment for PHN. About 15 percent of people who develop shingles have blisters in the eye area. A few of these people develop permanent vision deficits.

About one in three people will develop shingles during their lifetime. An estimated 500,000 to 1 million cases occur in the United States each year. People who live to age 85 have a 50 percent chance of developing shingles. Most people have only one outbreak, although repeat outbreaks are possible, especially in immunocompromised individuals.

Shingles is not contagious; it cannot be passed from person to person. However, if a person who has never had chickenpox or has not been vaccinated against the disease comes into direct contact with fluid from shingles blisters (e.g., a grandparent with shingles holding a child not vaccinated against chickenpox), that person may become infected and develop chickenpox.

Administration of Shingles Vaccine

Until 2017, there was only one shingles vaccine, Zostavax, approved for people over age 50 years in the United States. Zostavax contains the same live attenuated virus as varicella vaccine given to prevent chickenpox, except that the shingles vaccine is 14 times stronger than the dose given to immunize against chickenpox. In October 2017, a second shingles vaccine, Shingrix, was approved by the FDA and recommended by ACIP for adults over age 50. Shingrix is a recombinant subunit vaccine derived from genetically engineered Chinese hamster ovary cells. It requires two doses, the second two to six months after the first.

The original shingles vaccine, Zostavax, is just over 50 percent effective in preventing shingles, but it is 67 percent effective in preventing PHN. In clinical trials, Shingrix, was just over 90 percent effective in preventing shingles and reducing PHN for at least four years. As of 2018, the CDC was recommending revaccination with Shingrix for individuals who were originally vaccinated with Zostavax, as well as vaccination with Shingrix of all unvaccinated individuals over age 50 years.

Adverse Effects

Both shingles vaccines cause mild adverse effects. The most common are transient pain, swelling, itching, and redness at the injection site, and muscle ache or headache. A few people vaccinated with Zostavax develop a mild rash.

Special Populations

Certain medical situations may change the recommended administration of shingles vaccine. Individuals should discuss any conditions that may alter use of shingles vaccine with their physician.

- Zostavax contains gelatin and the antibiotic neomycin. People who have had a severe allergic reaction to either of these or other vaccine components or to chickenpox vaccine should not be vaccinated with Zostavax. Shingrix does not contain either antibiotics or gelatin.
- People who have diseases and disorders that compromise the immune system (e.g., HIV infection), are taking immune-suppressant drugs, have certain blood and lymph cancers, or are receiving chemotherapy

or radiation should not be vaccinated with Zostavax and should discuss advisability of vaccination with Shingrix with their physician.
- Moderately or severely ill individuals should wait until they are
  healthy to be vaccinated.
- Individuals who are certain they have never had chickenpox or have
  never received a vaccine against chickenpox should not be vaccinated.

What Makes This Vaccine Controversial?

Shingles vaccine is not controversial except for individuals who
reject all vaccines. However, many older people skip this vaccine or are
unaware of it.

Varicella (Chickenpox)

Varicella vaccine (Varivax) is a live attenuated vaccine that protects
against chickenpox, which is also called varicella. It is given either as a
single-antigen vaccine or as the four-combination vaccine MMRV (Pro-
Quad). The single-antigen vaccine has been available in the United States
since 1995 and the combination vaccine since 2005.

Chickenpox is caused by *varicella zoster* virus, the same virus that
causes shingles in older people. It is spread by breathing in respiratory
droplets expelled into the air through coughing and sneezing of an infected
person or by direct contact with broken pox blisters. If one infected person
is in a room with 100 unvaccinated individuals for several hours, about
85 unvaccinated people will contract chickenpox. Incubation time is generally 14–16 days. People are infectious two days before a rash appears.
If varicella vaccine is given within three days postexposure to the virus,
it is between 70 percent and 100 percent effective in preventing illness or
modifying the severity of symptoms.

Chickenpox causes a red rash that begins on the face and moves downward. Soon the rash develops into very itchy, fluid-filled blisters that cover
the body. Blisters can also form on the mucous membranes lining the airways and genitals. After four or five days, the blisters crust over. People
remain infectious until all blisters have formed a crust. Fever accompany-
ing chickenpox in children rarely goes above 102°F (38.8°C). Symptoms
are often more severe in adolescents and adults.

Before the advent of the varicella vaccine, about 4 million cases of
chickenpox occurred in the United States each year, accounting for
11,000 hospitalizations and 100 deaths. Ninety percent of children contracted the disease by age 10 years. By 2000, vaccination coverage had

reached 80 percent, and the disease caused fewer than 10 deaths annually. Worldwide, the prevalence of chickenpox depends on the extent of immunization programs. Almost all unimmunized people contract the disease.

Administration of Varicella Vaccine

Varicella vaccine is given to children on the same schedule as MMR and can be given at the same office visit. If not given at the same time, 30 days should pass before the second vaccine is administered. Both MMRV and single-antigen varicella are given subcutaneously. Children should receive the first dose between 12 and 15 months of age with the second dose between 4 and 6 years, although it can be given earlier. People over age 13 years, including adults who have not been vaccinated or had chickenpox, should receive two doses four to eight weeks apart.

Adverse Effects

Although allergic reaction can occur, serious reactions to varicella vaccine are rare. The most common adverse effects are soreness, redness, or swelling at the injection site, and low fever. About 4 percent of people develop a mild rash within three weeks of vaccination. Consult the information on MMR for information on adverse effects of MMRV.

Special Populations

Certain medical situations may change the recommended administration of varicella vaccine. Parents should discuss any conditions that may alter the administration of the vaccine with their child's pediatrician.

- Varicella vaccine contains gelatin and the antibiotic neomycin. People who have had a severe allergic reaction to either these or any other vaccine component should not be vaccinated.
- Vaccination may not be appropriate for people who are immunocompromised, are taking immune-suppressant drugs, have cancer, or are receiving chemotherapy or radiation.
- People who have recently received a blood product may need to wait to be vaccinated.
- Moderately or severely ill individuals should wait until they are healthy to be vaccinated.
- Pregnant women should wait until the birth of the child to be vaccinated.

What Makes This Vaccine Controversial?

Anti-vaccination parents feel vaccination against what is normally a mild childhood illness is unnecessary. They object to introducing a virus into the body that may later reactivate as shingles even though the same potential for reactivation exists if a child gets the chickenpox naturally. This controversy is discussed in Chapter 11.

VACCINES NOT ROUTINELY GIVEN IN THE UNITED STATES

Vaccines against rabies and tuberculosis are not part of the recommended vaccination schedule in the United States. These vaccines are routinely used in developing countries where rabies and tuberculosis are common. However, both vaccines are licensed for use in the United States and are of great value when administered to select populations.

Rabies

The vaccine against rabies is the most common vaccine administered to a select civilian and military population. Rabies is caused by a virus that attacks the central nervous system. For people who are not vaccinated, it is always fatal. Dogs, cats, ferrets, rabbits, skunks, raccoons, coyotes, foxes, and bats are all susceptible to rabies and can transfer it to humans. The virus is found in saliva and usually is transmitted by the bite of an infected animal. Once the virus enters the body, it travels along nerve cells until it reaches the brain and spinal cord where it reproduces and eventually destroys the nervous system. It can take weeks or months for diagnostic symptoms to appear. By the time they are obvious, nothing can be done to stop the progress of the disease. Initial symptoms are general—headache, fever, and fatigue—but as the virus increases in concentration, symptoms develop such as anxiety, confusion, and hallucinations, ending with the classic foaming at the mouth symptom, extreme fear of water, and death.

Rabies vaccine is used like any other vaccine to prevent someone from acquiring the disease. Individuals who receive pre-exposure vaccination include veterinarians, animal handlers, cave explorers (because bats live in caves and frequently carry rabies), and people who work in the manufacture of rabies vaccine or in research laboratories where the virus is studied. Others who might benefit from pre-exposure vaccination include people who work with wildlife in situations where they might encounter rabid wild animals, travelers, humanitarian aid workers in developing countries, and military personnel likely to be exposed to animals in parts of the world where rabies is common.

Rabies vaccine is also highly effective if given promptly after a person is exposed to the virus. This use is called postexposure prophylaxis. Postexposure prophylaxis is effective only because the rabies virus reproduces slowly. This gives the body the two weeks or so it needs to make enough antibodies to control the disease.

Only 55 cases of rabies have occurred in the United States since 1990, 90 percent of which developed from contact with wild animals, mostly bats. Nevertheless, somewhere between 16,000 and 39,000 Americans are vaccinated each year after being bitten by an animal that may have been rabid. The WHO estimates that the rabies causes about 50,000 deaths and that 10 million people receive postexposure prophylaxis each year, mostly in Africa, the Indian subcontinent, and Asia where packs of feral dogs are common.

Administration of Rabies Vaccine

Rabies vaccines (Imovert and RabAvert in the United States) are made from chemically inactivated virus and are delivered by intramuscular injection. Pre-exposure vaccination consists of three doses on days 0, 7, and 21 or 28. Pregnant women seeking pre-exposure vaccination should wait until the baby is born unless the risk of exposure to rabies outweighs the risk to the fetus.

Postexposure prophylaxis for people who have never been vaccinated consists of extensive wound cleansing, four doses of rabies vaccine on days 0, 3, 7, and 14, and a dose of human rabies immune globulin (HRIG) on day 0. The immunoglobulin provides short-term passive immunity until the body generates antibodies to create long-lasting active immunity. People who have been vaccinated within five years of exposure to rabies usually receive two doses of vaccine plus HRIG. Since rabies is a fatal disease, there is no controversy about the use of this vaccine. There are no age or health restrictions on who receives postexposure prophylaxis, and although serious allergic reactions are possible, death without vaccination is certain.

Tuberculosis

The Bacille Calmette-Guérin (BCG) vaccine, first tested in humans in 1921, is the oldest vaccine still in use today. It is used to prevent tuberculosis in individuals who are not already infected. Tuberculosis is an airborne contagious disease caused by the bacterium *Mycobacterium tuberculosis*. It is most common in areas where people live crowded together in conditions of poverty. The vaccine contains live attenuated bacteria. It does not protect against all strains that cause tuberculosis, especially drug-resistant strains. Observational studies suggest that overall effectiveness is about 50 percent, although for unknown reasons, effectiveness can range from almost completely ineffective to 80 percent effective in different geographic populations. Although tuberculosis is uncommon in the United States, the WHO estimates that between 8 million and 10 million cases of the disease develop worldwide every year, causing 1–2 million deaths.

Administration of BCG Vaccine

BCG vaccine is officially recommended in 180 countries, but not in the United States.

In countries where tuberculosis is common, the vaccine is routinely given to newborns and young children, as it can be given safely only to people who are not already infected. In the United States, the vaccine is used only rarely and on an individual basis after consultation with an expert on tuberculosis. It may be given as a protective measure to uninfected children who cannot be separated from adults with untreated or ineffectively treated tuberculosis and to individuals who work with tuberculosis patients.

Oddly, BCG has been found to be an effective treatment for early or noninvasive bladder cancer. The vaccine is injected directly into the bladder and allowed to remain there for several hours. The patient then urinates, but some BCG cells remain in the bladder. They appear to attract immune system cells to the area where they attach to and destroy cancer cells, although it is not clear why this happens.

BCG vaccine may also have other uses. In July 2018, researchers reported on an eight-year preliminary study in people with type 1 diabetes. They found that injections of BCG vaccine brought blood sugar levels of study participants down to near normal levels. Type 1 diabetes is an autoimmune disease in which the cells that make insulin, a chemical needed for cells in the body to use glucose (sugar), are attacked and destroyed. Researchers theorize that BCG vaccine in some way directs cells in to use glucose in the absence of insulin. Additional research is under way.

VACCINES GIVEN ONLY TO U.S. ARMED FORCES

As of 2018, new military recruits are given the same CDC-recommended vaccinations, boosters, and catch-up doses of vaccines recommended for the civilian population. In addition, select personnel are also immunized against smallpox, anthrax, and adenovirus. These vaccines are reserved for military members, some civilians attached to the military (e.g., overseas military contractors), and very occasionally civilians in high-risk occupations. Who is vaccinated depends on the branch of service and the occupational risk of the individual. In addition, many military members receive vaccines approved for both civilian and military travelers based on health risks likely to be encountered during their deployment (see Vaccines Given to Travelers later in the chapter).

Adenovirus

Fifty-two types of adenovirus cause a variety of respiratory, gastrointestinal, and other infections. The adenovirus vaccine protects against type 4 and type 17 viruses that cause acute respiratory disease and influenza-like symptoms, eye and other infections, and serious complications such as pneumonia. The vaccine is approved only for use by military personnel ages 17–50 years. Adenoviruses are likely to infect new recruits because of their close living quarters. Before immunization, up to 80 percent of trainees contracted the virus and at least 20 percent had symptoms serious enough to require hospitalization. A vaccine (now discontinued) was developed in 1956 and used until 1998. No vaccinations were done between 1998 and 2011, at which time the immunization program was resumed with a new vaccine.

Adenovirus type 4 and type 7 vaccine is a live attenuated vaccine given as two oral tablets, one for each type of virus. Adverse effects are generally mild and include headache, cold-like symptoms, abdominal pain, nausea, and diarrhea. About 1 percent of individuals develop a fever. Serious health problems developing within six months of vaccination, which may or may not be related to the vaccine, include pneumonia, blood in urine or stool, and inflammation of the gastrointestinal system.

Anthrax

Anthrax spores are ranked among the top 21st-century bioterrorism threats. They are relatively easy and inexpensive to produce, spread easily, and remain infective for decades. For this reason, anthrax vaccine is recommended for military personnel, researchers who work with the disease, and a few civilians who work with animals and animal hides. During the Persian Gulf War in 1991, about 150,000 American troops were given anthrax vaccine. In 1998, the program was expanded to service members working in high-risk areas and those involved in homeland defense.

Anthrax is caused by toxins released by the bacterium *Bacillus anthracis*. This bacterium forms long-lived spores. When grazing animals eat the spores, they develop into anthrax bacteria. Humans acquire the disease by contact with an infected animal. The bacteria usually enter through a break in the skin. This form of anthrax is called cutaneous anthrax, and it is most often contracted by people who handle wool or hides. It causes skin ulcers, fever, and fatigue. If untreated, it kills about 20 percent of those infected. Anthrax can also be acquired from eating raw or undercooked meat from an infected animal. This form of anthrax causes nausea, vomiting, and fever. It can also be fatal.

The military is primarily concerned with weaponized inhalation anthrax. If *B. anthracis* is inhaled, within a few days it causes severe breathing problems, shock, meningitis, and death. Anthrax in various forms has been used as a bioterrorism weapon since the 1930s, but the main threat comes from concentrated aerosolized anthrax, which is not so easy to produce, but is very easy to distribute.

Anthrax vaccine adsorbed (BioThrax) is a toxoid vaccine made by chemically inactivating the toxin produced by *B. anthracis*. The vaccine has been licensed in the United States since 1970. It is administered by intramuscular injection for pre-exposure immunization and subcutaneously for postexposure prophylaxis. Pre-exposure immunization consists of a primary series of three injections at day 0, 1 month, and 6 months followed by boosters at 6 and 12 months after the final primary injection series. Yearly boosters are recommended to sustain immunity. Postexposure prophylaxis is given at day 0, 2 weeks, and 4 weeks along with antibiotics. The effectiveness of postexposure prophylaxis in humans remains unclear because recommendations are based only on animal testing.

Serious allergic reactions occur less than once in every 100,000 doses, but milder adverse effects such as redness, soreness, and itching at the injection site; muscle aches; headaches; and fatigue are common. Pre-exposure vaccination should not be given to pregnant women, immunocompromised individuals, and others with certain allergies and health problems. Because of the seriousness of inhaled anthrax, there are few limitations on postexposure prophylaxis.

Smallpox

The military has a long history of involvement in the development and testing of vaccines. During the Revolutionary War, General George Washington recognized that the British had a significant manpower advantage because many of their soldiers had been variolated (a riskier predecessor to vaccination) against smallpox. As early as 1777, Washington ordered new recruits to be variolated, and the smallpox rate in the army dropped from 17 percent to 1 percent.

Smallpox kills about 30 percent of people who are infected. Routine civilian vaccination against smallpox ended in the United States in 1972 because the benefits no longer outweighed the risks. Smallpox was declared eradicated worldwide in 1980. Nevertheless, the U.S. military continued to vaccinate new recruits until 1984. Between 1984 and 1990, smallpox vaccination was intermittent because of vaccine shortages, and inoculation was temporarily discontinued from 1990 to December 2002 when, faced with the possibility of smallpox being used as a weapon of bioterrorism, vaccination resumed for medical response teams and troops deployed to high-risk areas.

Smallpox vaccine (ACAM2000) contains a live pox virus that is a close relative of the smallpox virus. The virus causes a much milder reaction than the smallpox virus, but it still activates the immune system to make antibodies against smallpox. Because smallpox vaccine contains live virus, vaccinated individuals can pass the virus to unvaccinated people for several weeks after vaccination. Special care of the inoculation site must be taken during this time and certain activities are restricted.

Special training is required for doctors before they are allowed to handle smallpox vaccine. The vaccine is given by a process called scarification. A drop of vaccine is inserted with a two-pronged needle under the skin of the upper arm but not deep enough to cause bleeding. The site becomes red, itchy, and bumpy, and most people develop a fever. The scarification site must be kept covered and completely dry until the scab that forms drops off and new skin covers the site (2–4 weeks). Contact with the site or with bandages and clothing that have been in contact with the site can spread the virus to unimmunized people. Clothing and bedding that may have been in contact with the scarification site must be washed separately. There are other restrictions on activities (e.g., swimming, handling infants).

Rash, fever, and head and body aches are common adverse effects. Very serious and sometimes permanent adverse effects include myocarditis and pericarditis (infection of the heart muscle and surrounding membranes), encephalitis, severe skin infections, and blindness. People who are immunocompromised or have heart disease should not be vaccinated. People who have had eczema or atopic dermatitis are at higher risk for serious side effects. The vaccine has not been studied in pregnant or breastfeeding women. As of 2018, only select military personnel were vaccinated against smallpox, but the Department of Defense claims to have enough vaccine stockpiled to immunize most Americans in case of a bioterrorism emergency.

VACCINATIONS GIVEN TO TRAVELERS

Certain vaccines called geographic niche vaccines are given only to civilians and military personnel who visit or live in specific locations. Recommendations vary depending on the location, length of stay, and health of the traveler. The CDC tracks disease prevalence and worldwide traveler health requirements in a publication called the *Yellow Book*. This information is available online at the CDC's Travelers' Health website at https://wwwnc.cdc.gov/travel.

The Travelers' Health website allows individuals to enter their destination, information on their stay, and any special health considerations they have (e.g., pregnant, immunocompromised, travelling with children). The site then provides up-to-date information about required and recommended vaccines and health warnings for the chosen location. The WHO also maintains information on current disease outbreaks at http://www.who.int/csr/don/en.

Geographic niche vaccines are discussed in the chapter, but disease risk can change rapidly. Travelers are urged to check these websites well in advance of travel for the most recent information. Some vaccines require multiple doses over several weeks to create strong immunity, so travelers should take the timing of inoculations into consideration when planning travel.

Cholera

Cholera is an intestinal infection caused by the bacterium *Vibrio cholera*. It is transmitted by the oral–fecal route through contaminated food and water. It can also be contracted by eating raw or undercooked shellfish (e.g., raw oysters) mainly from the Gulf of Mexico, although this route of infection is uncommon. Cholera is almost never passed directly from person to person.

Cholera is rare in the United States and most developed countries. It thrives in crowded and unsanitary conditions such as slums and refugee camps where there is inadequate treatment of water and sewage. Outbreaks often occur after natural disasters such as hurricanes and tsunamis during which water supplies become contaminated with untreated sewage.

In 2017, a cholera epidemic developed in Syria and Yemen as a consequence of war. Attacks on water and sewage treatment plants resulted in contaminated water, and more than 475 attacks on medical facilities left most people unable to get treatment. It was estimated that at the height of the outbreak, 5,000 new cases of cholera occurred in Yemen each day. In 2017, the Democratic Republic of the Congo also experienced a cholera epidemic on par with that of Yemen and Syria because of internal warfare. Worldwide, researchers estimate there are between 1.4 million and 4.3 million cases of cholera each year accounting for between 28,000 and 142,000 deaths.

About 80 percent of people infected with *V. cholera* show no symptoms. Of those who do develop symptoms, the majority (up to 80 percent) have only mild to moderate illness. The remaining people develop severe, life-threatening symptoms. In severe illness, people produce copious amounts of watery diarrhea along with vomiting. Fluids can be lost at the rate of one quart (1 L) per hour, causing fatal dehydration, especially among infants, young children, pregnant women, and the elderly. Cholera can be treated successfully with rehydration fluids.

In 2016, the FDA licensed the first vaccine in the United States for the prevention of cholera. The vaccine, Vaxchora, is a live attenuated oral vaccine. A single dose given at least 10 days before travel to a region where cholera is common was found in clinical trials to be 90–93 percent effective. Before this, two WHO-approved oral cholera vaccines (Dukoral and ShanChol) were available in many other countries to immunize people over age two years. Dukoral contains heat and chemically killed bacteria and a subunit protein of the bacterial toxin. ShanChol contains whole-killed bacteria. Both vaccines can cause headaches, fatigue, and fever and require two doses. These vaccines are only 50–60 percent effective. Children under age two years, pregnant women, and immunocompromised individuals should not be vaccinated. For most travelers, the risk of contracting cholera is low. Risk can be further reduced by good hygiene practices, boiling water, and avoiding raw foods including unpeeled fruits and raw vegetables.

Japanese Encephalitis

Japanese encephalitis is caused by a *flavivirus* and is spread by the bite of an infected mosquito. Risk of contracting the disease is greatest for individuals spending an extended period in parts of rural Asia. The vaccine is given mainly to military personnel and people such as missionaries and humanitarian aid workers who will be working in rural areas. Tourists visiting major Asian cities and staying less than one month are unlikely to contract the disease.

Japanese encephalitis virus causes fever, stiff neck, nausea, and vomiting. Symptoms appear about two weeks after the individual is infected. Some people go on to develop encephalitis. About 25 percent of people who progress to encephalitis die and another 50 percent are left with permanent disabilities.

The Japanese encephalitis vaccine (IXIARO in the United States, JESPECT in Europe and Australia) contains chemically inactivated virus and cannot cause the disease. A live attenuated vaccine is used in China. The vaccine is recommended for travelers over age two months who will be staying in rural locations where the disease is common. It is given as a series of two shots 28 days apart. People over age 17 may receive a booster after one year. Adverse effects are generally mild and include headaches and body aches and fatigue. About 1 percent of people develop soreness at the injection site.

Typhoid

Typhoid fever, also known as enteric fever, is caused by *Salmonella typhi* bacteria. People acquire the bacteria through contaminated food and water. Typhoid causes a high fever, intense stomach pain, tenderness and abdominal distension, headache, fatigue, weakness, and sometimes a rash. If left untreated, about 30 percent of people die. Increasingly, some strains of typhoid are antibiotic resistant, complicating treatment even when high-quality medical care is available.

About 3 percent of people who recover from typhoid become carriers of the disease. They can infect other people even though they have no symptoms themselves. The most famous carrier is Mary Mallon (1869–1938), known as Typhoid Mary. In the early 1900s, she infected more than 50 people in New York City.

In areas where typhoid infection is common, travelers can avoid the disease by drinking only bottled water, avoiding uncooked foods, and peeling fruits and raw vegetables. Vaccination is only 50–80 percent effective, so even if vaccinated, individuals must be careful about what they consume. Typhoid is rare in the United States. About 80 percent of cases in the United States occur in people who have travelled to Mexico or developing countries in Asia, South America, and Africa. Typhoid is especially common in rural and nontourist areas where water and sewage treatment are limited and in areas where natural disasters have contaminated the water supply with untreated sewage. Worldwide, about 22 million people contract the disease each year and between 200,000 and 600,000 die.

Vaccination is suggested for only for responders to natural disasters and people living in high-risk areas for six weeks or more. People in close contact with a typhoid carrier and those working in laboratories with *S. typhi* are also vaccinated.

Yellow Fever

Yellow fever is caused by a *flavivirus* transmitted by several species of *Aedes* and *Haemagogus* mosquitoes found in Africa, Central America, and South America. Flaviviruses also cause Japanese encephalitis, dengue fever, tick-borne encephalitis, and Zika virus disease. Yellow fever causes influenza-like symptoms—fever, chills, head and body aches, nausea, and fatigue. In about 20 percent of infected individuals, the disease progresses to severe symptoms including liver damage, severe bleeding, multiorgan failure, and death. There is no specific treatment. A list of countries where yellow fever is common can be found at https://wwwnc .cdc.gov/travel/yellowbook/2016/infectious-diseases-related-to-travel/ yellow-fever#4728.

Yellow fever vaccine (YF-Vax) is a live attenuated vaccine given subcutaneously. The vaccine is almost 100 percent effective. The CDC reports only 23 failures in more than 540 million doses. As of June 2016, a single dose of the vaccine was regarded as providing lifelong immunity. Before this date, a booster was required every 10 years. International health regulations allow countries to demand proof of immunization against yellow fever for entry into the country, and some may be slow to lift the 10-year booster requirement. International travelers should check the entry requirements of the countries they plan to visit.

Yellow fever vaccine is suitable for all individuals over age nine months traveling to places where the disease is found or working with the virus in the laboratory or a manufacturing facility. Mild effects include headache, muscle ache, and low fever. Pregnant women, immunocompromised individuals, and people severely allergic to eggs (the virus is grown in chicken eggs), gelatin, or any other component of the vaccine should not be vaccinated. Severe allergic reactions occur less than once in one million doses.

VACCINES NOT USED IN THE UNITED STATES

Each country has its own vaccine approval process that aims to balance vaccine risks with the needs of its population based on the prevalence of each vaccine-preventable disease and the effectiveness of the vaccine. The result is that not all vaccines are available in all countries. There are several reasons for this.

- A disease is so rare in a particular country that there is no need to vaccinate against it.
- Regulatory agencies have decided the vaccine is not adequately effective to justify licensing it.
- Regulatory agencies feel the adverse effects of the vaccine outweigh its benefits.
- Regulatory agencies want more information about the vaccine and the conditions of its production before it is licensed.

Dengue

In December 2015, Sanofi Pasteur, the vaccines division of the French company Sanofi, announced that it had received authorization in Mexico to market Dengvaxia, the world's first vaccine against dengue fever. Approvals in Brazil, the Philippines, and El Salvador followed quickly, and by the end of 2017, 22 countries had approved the vaccine.

Dengue fever, also called breakbone fever, is caused by four related strains of a *flavivirus*. It is transmitted from person to person by the bite of infected *Aedes* mosquitoes. The disease is found in about 100 tropical and subtropical countries including Caribbean islands such as Puerto Rico. In the past, outbreaks have occurred in the Southeastern United States and in Hawaii.

Five to seven days after becoming infected, an individual develops a fever, severe headache, body and joint aches, and a rash. After this, patients appear to improve, but some people relapse and develop dengue hemorrhagic fever. With dengue hemorrhagic fever, the blood vessels become permeable. Fluid enters the tissues causing hypotension (low blood pressure) that can lead to potentially fatal shock. Other symptoms include internal bleeding indicated by bloody vomit and bloody stool. There is no specific treatment for dengue, but individuals who survive gradually improve. Every year, about 220 million people contract dengue fever. Of those, about two million people, mostly children, develop severe cases with bleeding complications and many die.

The dengue vaccine is a live attenuated recombinant DNA vaccine that protects against four strains of the virus. Immunity to one strain does not provide immunity to other strains. The vaccine is licensed for use in people ages 9–54 years. Complete immunization requires three doses, the second given 6 months after the first and the third 12 months after the first. The vaccine is about 65 percent effective in preventing dengue fever in people over age 9 years and 93 percent effective in preventing cases serious enough to require hospitalization in this age group. However, post licensure, the vaccine was found to cause serious adverse effects for some individuals.

In November 2017, the WHO advised that the vaccine should be used only in places where there is substantial dengue present and where at least 70 percent of the target population have antibodies against at least one strain of dengue virus. WHO vaccine experts concluded from postlicensure data that risk of severe dengue requiring hospitalization was significantly increased among vaccinated individuals who had not already made antibodies against at least one strain of dengue at the time of vaccination. This adverse effect was discovered when 830,000 children, many of whom had never had dengue fever, were vaccinated in the Philippines. On later becoming infected with a different strain, some of these vaccinated children became severely ill. As a result, the government of the Philippines stopped the vaccination program and forced the manufacturer to recall the vaccine from the Philippines and set stricter limits on its use. An evaluation of this complication is ongoing, but as of early 2018, other countries were reevaluating their dengue vaccination programs.

Ebola Virus Disease

Ebola viruses belong to a family of viruses that cause hemorrhagic fevers characterized by vomiting, gastrointestinal bleeding, bleeding from mucous membranes, headaches, muscle aches, tissue swelling, low blood pressure, and fever. The death rate ranges from 25 percent to 90 percent, depending on the species of Ebola virus. Five species had been identified as of early 2018, four of which cause serious disease in humans.

Many animals, including monkeys, chimpanzees, gorillas, fruit bats, forest antelope, and porcupines, can be infected with Ebola. The virus is transmitted to humans by contact with blood, secretions, and organs of an infected animal. Once in the human population, the virus spreads from person to person by contact with blood and body secretions. It can also be spread by contact with bedding, clothing, or other surfaces contaminated with these fluids, making containment difficult. Small, sporadic outbreaks of Ebola virus disease have occurred in Africa for many years. The most widespread outbreak as of early 2018 occurred in Guinea, Liberia, and Sierra Leone and lasted from March 2014 until December 2015. At least 11,000 people died.

In May 2018, the Democratic Republic Congo approved an Ebola vaccine known as rVSV-ZEBOV developed by the Public Health Agency of Canada and NewLink Genetics and manufactured by Merck Vaccines USA. It is a live attenuated recombinant vector vaccine genetically engineered to stimulate antibodies against *Ebolavirus zaire,* the species that caused most of the illness in the 2014 outbreak. This vaccine was used successfully to contain a small outbreak of Ebola in the Congo that began in May 2018.

Another Ebola vaccine, cAd3-ZEBOV, developed by GlaxoSmith-Kline, appeared highly effective and as of mid-2018 was in Phase III trials. This is a recombinant vector vaccine derived from a chimpanzee virus genetically engineered to stimulate antibody production against *E. zaire* and *E. sudan.*

Kyasanur Forest Disease

Kyasanur Forest disease (KFD), also called monkey fever or monkey disease, is a tick-borne hemorrhagic viral disease caused by a *flavivirus.* The disease is found mainly in Karnataka state on the west coast of India where it is spread by at least 15 species of ticks. Between 400 and 500 cases are reported every year, mostly in people who live or work in forested areas and have contact with monkeys.

Symptoms of KFD include fever, severe headache, severe pain in the arms and legs, low blood pressure, sore throat, diarrhea, vomiting, inability to eat, and insomnia. About one week after these symptoms appear, bleeding symptoms begin. Individuals bleed from the nose, vomit blood, and have bloody stool. The death rate is 3–5 percent. About 10–20 percent of those who recover have relapses that include mental confusion, tremors, vision problems, and fever. The vaccine against KFD is an example of a highly local niche vaccine. It is available only in India and is only given to at-risk people in a limited geographic area.

Leptospirosis

Leptospirosis is a disease of humans and animals caused by multiple strains of the spirochete bacterium *Leptospira interrogans.* It is the most common zoonotic disease in the world. Leptospirosis can be acquired through breaks in the skin when in direct contact with an infected animal or its fluids or feces or through contaminated soil or water. The bacterium can also be inhaled and enter the body through the mucous membranes of the respiratory system. Person-to-person transmission is rare. Carriers of the disease include rodents and almost all domestic animals—cattle, sheep, horses, goats, swine, buffalo, and dogs. People at highest risk are those who work closely with animals. Outbreaks also can occur after natural disasters in which there is flooding. The disease was found in dogs relocated to Florida after hurricane Marie decimated Puerto Rico in 2017.

Symptoms of leptospirosis mimic those of many other diseases, and diagnostic testing is not easily available. Consequently, the disease is considered seriously underreported. Estimates based on testing blood for antibodies against *L. interrogans* concluded that 80 percent of people living in the tropics encounter the disease during their lifetime. Prevalence in nontropical areas tends to correlate to the size of the rat population, since rats are common urban carriers of the bacteria.

Leptospirosis causes a fever of 100.5–104°F (38–40°C). Most people have influenza-like symptoms, pain behind the eyes, sensitivity to light, nausea, and vomiting. Between 5 percent and 15 percent of infected individuals develop serious complications such as jaundice, liver damage, kidney damage, bleeding from the lungs, and systemic shock. Leptospirosis is treated with antibiotics.

No WHO-recommended human vaccines are available against leptospirosis, but human vaccines are available in Cuba and China. A vaccine for dogs is available in the United States. Its use is controversial since immunity lasts only one year, and it protects against only four strains of the bacterium.

Plague

Plague, known as the Black Death, killed between 75 million and 200 million people during an outbreak in the 1300s in Europe. Today, plague is still a serious disease with a mortality rate of 60 percent in untreated individuals. Prompt treatment with antibiotics substantially reduces the chance of death.

Plague is caused by *Yersinia pestis* bacteria. It is a zoonotic disease. *Y. pestis* infects small rodents such as rats and ground squirrels. A flea bites an infected animal and becomes infected. The infected flea then bites a human and transfers *Y. pestis* to the human. Plague can also be acquired through direct contact with the fluids from an infected animal or by inhaling respiratory droplets of an infected animal or person. In 2017, a major plague outbreak occurred in Madagascar, sickening more than 1,800 people and killing at least 143.

Three to seven days after being infected, the individual develops a sudden high fever, chills, head and body aches, abdominal pain, nausea, vomiting and general weakness. There are three forms of plague. Bubonic plague (the Black Death of the Middle Ages) develops from the bite of an infected flea causing inflamed painful lymph nodes called buboes. In time, the skin turns black. Septicemia plague develops from flea bites or direct contact with infected fluids. The infection spreads through the bloodstream without forming buboes. Pneumatic plague develops in the lungs from inhaling respiratory droplets containing *Y. pestis*. It is the rarest and most deadly form of plague and is considered a potential weapon of bioterrorism.

Plague occurs rarely in the United States and is usually confined to the Southwest. On average, only three cases are reported each year. However, in 2015, 15 cases and 4 deaths were reported, several of which were linked to a campground in Yosemite National Park in California. Worldwide, plague is found in all continents except Antarctica. The 1,000–2,000 cases that are reported to the WHO each year are considered a substantial undercount. In mid-2017, researchers in the United States announced successful trials of a new plague vaccine that could be added to rodent bait. Preventing plague in animals substantially reduces the chance of transmission to humans. Lacing bait with vaccine is the same strategy used to control the spread of rabies in wildlife.

Researchers have been trying to develop an effective human vaccine against plague since 1890. In the past, a vaccine was available in the United States. The vaccine was not very effective and caused unacceptable adverse effects, so its use was discontinued. Canada allows the use of plague vaccine very sparingly for people at high risk of exposure. The vaccine requires multiple doses and boosters to remain effective, and it causes substantial adverse effects. Because of the potential for *Y. pestis* to be used as a bioterrorism weapon, research is ongoing to develop an effective human plague vaccine.

Polio Vaccine–Oral

OPV was used in the United States for many years until it was replaced by IPV in 2000. OPV is approved by the WHO and is the vaccine of choice in many countries because of its ease of administration. It is a live attenuated vaccine. See Polio Vaccine–Inactivated above for symptoms of poliomyelitis.

Originally OPV was formulated to provide immunity against all strains of *poliovirus*—type 1, type 2, and type 3. However, the type 2 strain has been eradicated. In a massive worldwide effort by the Global Polio Eradication Initiative, all OPV containing live attenuated type 2 virus was required to be destroyed by boiling, bleaching, or burying in concrete containers in the two-week period between April 17, 2016, and May 1, 2016, after which only the new, two-strain OPV was to be used. By omitting the type 2 virus, OPV is more effective against types 1 and 3, and the chance of mutation of the type 2 strain into a variant that could cause serious illness has been eliminated.

The WHO recommends a three-dose series of OPV beginning as early as six weeks of age, with four weeks between doses. The WHO also recommends an additional dose of IPV at 14 weeks. This can be given simultaneously with the third dose of OPV. In countries where polio is present, a dose of OPV at birth is recommended, followed by the standard series. Many countries, however, have alternate schedules based on the needs of their population.

OPV is more effective at stimulating immunity than IPV. One dose of OPV creates immunity in almost half of the recipients. Three doses provide almost 100 percent coverage, and immunity is lifelong.

Because OPV contains live attenuated virus, it can in rare cases (1 in 2.4 million doses) cause a serious adverse event called vaccine-associated paralytic poliomyelitis (VAPP). VAPP is believed to occur when the attenuated virus spontaneously mutates into a more virulent form that can cause paralytic polio. The risk of this occurring is greatest with the first dose and is most likely to occur in immunocompromised children. According to the Polio Global Eradication Initiative, during the first six months of 2018, 15 cases of vaccine-associated polio were reported worldwide—6 in the Democratic Republic of the Congo, 5 in Somalia, 2 in Nigeria, and 1 in Papua New Guinea. This compares with 13 cases of naturally acquired polio during the same period. Naturally acquired polio occurred only in Afghanistan and Pakistan.

A side effect of OPV is that live polio virus are shed in stool for up to six weeks after vaccination. Unvaccinated individuals who are exposed to virus-contaminated stool can develop polio, although many develop only mild cases and then have lifelong immunity. This feature helps support herd immunity.

Q Fever

Q fever is caused by the bacterium *Coxiella burnetii*. It is one of the world's most infectious organisms. Half of all people infected with a single *C. burnetii* bacterium will develop Q fever. The disease was first recognized in humans in Australia in 1935, but it is found worldwide, including in most of the United States and Canada. Cattle, sheep, and goats can be infected. Humans become infected when they are exposed to fluids from infected animals. Ticks can also transmit the disease to humans; however, most people become infected by inhaling the bacterium.

Symptoms of Q fever vary substantially from person to person. About half of all people show no symptoms while others have mild influenza-like symptoms. A minority of people develop severe illness with a fever of 104–105°F (40–40.5°C), head and body aches, cough, vomiting, diarrhea, and chest pains. Complications can include pneumonia, hepatitis, myocarditis (inflammation of heart tissue), and miscarriage or preterm delivery.

Q fever can be treated with antibiotics. Less than 2 percent of hospitalized patients die. *C. burnetii* can remain in the body for long periods and in some people, especially those who are immunocompromised, trigger complications that develop months later.

Q fever became a reportable disease in the United States in 1999. One hundred and fifty-six cases were reported in 2015, with dairy and slaughterhouse workers at highest risk. Nevertheless, this is likely a major undercount since many people develop few or no symptoms. Q fever outbreaks tend to be regional. Between 2007 and 2014, 4,000 cases were reported in the Netherlands. Other recent outbreaks have occurred in Afghanistan and Iraq and have affected U.S. military personnel stationed there.

The Q fever vaccine (Q-VAX) contains chemically killed whole bacteria that have been grown in chicken eggs. It is given as a single subcutaneous injection. Before receiving the vaccine, it is *essential* that the individual have a skin test to determine if he or she already has antibodies to Q fever. The vaccine *cannot* be given to people who have already had Q fever, who have already received the vaccine, or who have antibodies to Q fever as indicated by the skin test. People who meet any of these three conditions and who receive the vaccine are at high risk for severe adverse reactions. In people who can safely receive the vaccine, about half have redness and soreness at the injections site and about 9 percent develop a headache.

Tick-Borne Encephalitis

Tick-borne encephalitis (TBE) is caused by three subtypes of a *flavivirus* that are related to the viruses that cause dengue fever, Japanese encephalitis, yellow fever, and Zika virus disease. The three subtypes are designated European, Siberian, and Far Eastern. The Far Eastern subtype causes the most severe illness and the most permanent disabilities. TBE is common in wooded parts of central Europe, Russia, countries that were once part of the Soviet Union, and parts of China. The disease is transmitted from small mammals to humans by ticks. In humans, it causes high fever, nausea, and vomiting, and can attack the central nervous system and cause paralysis and permanent neurological damage. An estimated 10,000 people are hospitalized with TBE each year.

Immunization against TBE is part of the recommended vaccination schedule in many countries where the disease is common. The vaccines (FSME-IMMUN and Encepur with two other vaccines produced in Russia and one in China) contain inactivated virus that provide cross-protection against all three subtypes in children and adults. The recommended age and the number of doses for complete immunization varies across countries and vaccine manufacturers, but in all cases, multiple doses across a minimum of six months are required along with regular booster shots to maintain immunity. TBE vaccine is not available in the United States, but FSME-IMMUN is licensed for use in adults in Canada.

As indicated in this chapter, no vaccine is 100 percent free of side effects, although almost all are mild and transitory. Likewise, although vaccines are highly effective in preventing disease, they are not 100 percent effective in every individual. When developing vaccine recommendations, governmental medical agencies consider the age at which the individual is most vulnerable to the vaccine-preventable disease and must balance risks and benefits of vaccination based on the severity of the disease, its prevalence in the population, economic costs of both the vaccine and the disease, and frequency and severity of adverse effects.

Most vaccines cause mild adverse effects including transient redness, swelling, and pain at the injection site, low fever, and mild headache and muscle ache. Moderate effects include high fever and transient febrile convulsions. Serious adverse effects are extremely rare but include anaphylaxis, encephalitis, permanent neurological damage, coma, and death.

Immunocompromised individuals are more likely than healthy individuals to experience adverse events. In some cases, these individuals should not be vaccinated because the health risk outweighs the benefit. Individuals should always be informed of the potential risks of receiving the vaccine (required by law in the United States) and should share with their health care provider any medical conditions and drugs, herbs, supplements, or other treatments that may influence the outcome of vaccination.

CHAPTER 6

History of Vaccine Resistance

The very first vaccinations were against smallpox. Smallpox was common and highly contagious. It killed 80–90 percent of infants and 20–30 percent of anyone else who became infected. Of those who recovered, about one-third were left with facial scars or permanent disabilities. One might think that a vaccine to prevent such a hazardous disease would be met with universal acclaim and enthusiasm. It was not. From the first vaccine against smallpox to the recent one against human papillomavirus, there have been people opposed to vaccination.

The strength of the anti-vaccination movement has varied over the past 225 years. When the prevalence of a vaccine-preventable disease is low, vaccine resistance tends to rise. When outbreaks of a vaccine-preventable disease occur, vaccine refusal tends to fall. Today, the vaccine debate remains active in many countries.

EARLY OPPOSITION

English physician Edward Jenner (1749–1823) is credited with discovering a method of vaccinating people against smallpox in 1796, but before that, many cultures used a method called variolation to create immunity to the disease. There are two strains of smallpox virus, *Variola major,* which is often deadly, and *Variola minor,* which causes much milder cases. Variolation worked by transferring material from the scab of someone with a mild case of smallpox to another individual who would then develop mild illness but acquire permanent immunity to the deadlier smallpox strain. The success of variolation depended heavily on choosing smallpox material from a person who had disease caused by *Variola minor* and weakening this material further by exposing it to air.

Variolation was not without risk. Variolated individuals were contagious for several weeks and had to be kept away from people who did not already have immunity. In addition, 1 to 2 percent of variolated individuals developed serious cases of smallpox and died. At a time when there was no treatment for smallpox, a 2 percent risk of death seemed acceptable when compared to the death and disability rate from naturally contracting the disease.

The first written record of variolation appears in Chinese literature dating from 1549, but almost certainly the technique had been used for centuries. The Chinese variolated by grinding dried smallpox scabs into a powder and puffing the powder through a tube into the nose of an uninfected person. In parts of Africa, parents wrapped a cloth around the arm of an infected child and then transferred the cloth to a child who was not immune with the expectation of inducing mild illness. This procedure continued in Sudan until around 1900.

Variolation came to England by way of Turkey. Lady Mary Wortley Montagu (1689–1762), wife of the British ambassador, was introduced to the procedure during their time in Constantinople. She was so impressed that she had her young son variolated by Charles Maitland, a physician attached to the British embassy. The Montagus and Maitland returned to England in 1718. When a smallpox epidemic ravaged London several years later, Lady Montagu asked the physician to variolate her daughter.

Maitland invited other doctors to witness the procedure. Initially, doctors were skeptical, but Lady Montagu persuaded Caroline, wife of King George II, to allow Maitland to perform variolation on six prisoners in Newgate Prison who were scheduled to be hanged. Each man was variolated and later exposed to smallpox with the condition that if he survived, he would be released. A few weeks later, six healthy men walked away from their death sentences. After that, the royal family had some of their children variolated, and the procedure gained public acceptance. At this time, variolation was completely voluntary, and there was no outcry against the procedure.

Opposition in America

Word of variolation spread to the American colonies in the early 1700s, but unlike in England, the procedure caused furious controversy. Cotton

Mather (1663–1728), a Puritan minister in Boston, discovered that his slave, Onesimus, had been variolated as a child in Africa. When a smallpox epidemic broke out in Boston in 1721, Mather had his son variolated and encouraged others to follow his example.

Outcry against the procedure was immediate. Most Boston doctors vigorously opposed variolation as did many religious leaders and members of the public. Opponents argued that the procedure was unnatural, spread smallpox, made the individual susceptible to other diseases, and could be fatal. There was some truth to these arguments. Variolation could spread blood-borne diseases such as syphilis, and variolated individuals were briefly contagious and could spread smallpox if not quarantined.

Cotton Mather did not attempt to perform variolation himself, but he actively promoted the procedure in pamphlets and by preaching that inoculation was a gift from God. Mather could find only one doctor in Boston, Zabidel Boylston (1679–1766), who was willing to perform variolations. The variolation debate became so heated that Mather's house was firebombed by anti-variolationists. By the end of the 1721 epidemic, 5,889 Bostonians had contracted smallpox, resulting in 844 deaths. Only 17 variolated individuals died, but that did not change the minds of the anti-variolationists.

George Washington Supports Variolation

It took the Revolutionary War (1775–1783) and the leadership of George Washington to overcome objections to variolation in America. Washington, who had survived smallpox as a teenager, concluded that the disease threatened the effectiveness of the army. He demanded that soldiers be variolated. This was the first attempt to impose mandatory inoculation. Washington's demand was opposed by the Continental Congress, which specifically forbade military variolation. Its objections were the same as those in Boston 55 years earlier.

In early 1777, Washington used his political influence to oust the anti-variolation head of the military medical service and replace him with a pro-variolation physician. He then ignored Congress, quietly variolated soldiers in small groups, and sent them to secret isolation centers in private homes and churches until they were no longer contagious. No smallpox epidemic occurred, and the following year, the death rate from smallpox in the troops dropped from 17 percent to 1 percent. When the war was over and variolated soldiers returned home, they were living proof to their families and neighbors of the success of the procedure.

THE FIRST TRUE VACCINATION

Variolation or contracting natural smallpox and surviving were the only ways to acquire immunity to the disease until 1796 when Edward Jenner (1749–1823) discovered how to intentionally use cowpox to prevent smallpox. Cowpox is a mild disease that causes pus-filled blisters on the udders of cows and can be transferred to the hands and arms of people exposed to these blisters. For years, farmers had observed that people who got cowpox did not get smallpox, although they could not explain why. Today we know that cowpox and smallpox viruses are so closely related that infection with cowpox virus stimulates the formation of antibodies against the smallpox virus.

Jenner, who was variolated as a child, grew up in rural England. He knew of the folk wisdom that said cowpox protected against smallpox. After training as a physician in London and Scotland, he returned to the countryside to practice medicine. There he developed the idea that the protection cowpox provided could not only be spread from cows to humans but could be transferred from person to person. He tested this idea by taking pus from the cowpox blister of a young woman and scratching it into the arm of an eight-year-old boy. The boy became mildly ill with a low fever, but within two weeks was completely healthy. Jenner then inoculated the boy with fluid from a fresh smallpox blister. The boy remained healthy even after Jenner exposed him to smallpox a second time. Jenner called the procedure vaccination from the Latin *vacca,* meaning cow.

People did not die from cowpox, which made the procedure much safer than variolation with its up to 2 percent death rate. Despite this, cowpox inoculation was opposed by the same forces that opposed variolation in Colonial America—doctors and religious leaders. Doctors objected for economic reasons. Variolation provided a steady income. Acquiring cowpox infection from either a cow or another person was easy and often free. Religious leaders claimed that God sent disease as punishment and that vaccination interfered with God's will. Newspapers ridiculed the idea of a cow disease protecting humans from illness. One popular cartoon published in 1802 showed cow heads popping out of various body parts of people who had been vaccinated.

In 1797, Jenner submitted a paper on vaccination to the Royal Society, which rejected it for publication. He performed vaccinations on more individuals and eventually self-published a pamphlet about his results. He also actively recruited other physicians to perform cowpox vaccinations and supplied them with the vaccine. By 1800, cowpox vaccination had spread across Europe. Variolation gradually fell into disuse as people became more familiar with the safer cowpox vaccine.

ANTI-VACCINATIONISTS ORGANIZE AGAINST BRITISH LAWS

By 1840, the British government had become active in passing legislation to protect public health. The Vaccination Act of 1840 made variolation illegal and provided free cowpox vaccinations for the poor. Some taxpayers objected to paying for the poor to be vaccinated, but the procedure was voluntary and did not spark significant public protest.

The Vaccine Act of 1853, however, had a major impact on public opinion. This Act made infant vaccination mandatory in England and Wales. Parents who failed to comply could be fined or imprisoned. The 1853 Act was the first British attempt at legislating compulsory vaccination. Compared to other countries in Europe, Parliament was behind the times. Denmark, Sweden, Bavaria, and several other German states had passed compulsory vaccination laws 35 years earlier.

The Vaccine Act of 1853 was poorly received by the public. The British Anti-Vaccination League was formed to protest the law. The League printed pamphlets against vaccination and led violent anti-vaccination demonstrations in at least half a dozen towns. As a result, although compulsory vaccination was officially the law, the law was only sporadically enforced.

A similar Act in 1867 increased the age of mandatory vaccination to 14 years. In response, the Anti-Compulsory Vaccination League was founded. Vaccine resistance grew stronger. The main argument against compulsory vaccination was that it restricted personal liberty and gave the government control over an individual's body. Enforcement of the 1853 and 1867 Acts was delegated to local officials. Strong public resistance and the anti-vaccination beliefs of many of these officials resulted in lax enforcement. Parents who chose not to vaccinate were rarely punished.

Enforcement procedures changed dramatically in 1871 when laws were passed that punished not just vaccine-refusing parents but also any local official who failed to enforce compulsory vaccination. Vigorous forced vaccination only fanned the flames of resistance. Anti-vaccination pamphlets and journals circulated among the well educated, while marches and sometimes violent protests drew working-class vaccine opponents. In March 1885, the Leicester Demonstration March, complete with anti-vaccination signs, a child's coffin, and an effigy of Edward Jenner, claimed to have drawn between 80,000 and 100,000 people from across England, although modern research suggests the number was much smaller.

In response to pressure from anti-vaccinationists, Parliament established a committee to study vaccination. The committee concluded that vaccination did protect against smallpox but that parents should be allowed a conscientious objector exemption and fines for noncompliance should be dropped. These provisions were incorporated into the Vaccination Act of 1898, effectively ending the first attempt at compulsory vaccination in Britain.

RESPONSE TO VOLUNTARY VACCINATION

One year after the Vaccine Act of 1898 authorized a conscientious objector exemption to vaccination, the Second Boer War (1899–1902) broke out between the British Empire and the Boer Republics of Transvaal and the Orange Free State in South Africa. The British military, not bound by the 1898 Act, required soldiers headed to Africa to be vaccinated against typhoid. There was strong public resistance to this requirement, and typhoid vaccine allegedly was dumped off ships into the harbor at Southampton in protest. Eventually, the military gave in to public pressure and made vaccination of British soldiers voluntary. Ninety-five percent refused the vaccine because of fear, public opinion, and its unpleasant side effects.

The results were disastrous. Arthur Conan Doyle (1859–1930), author of the Sherlock Holmes stories and a retired physician, volunteered for three months at a hospital in South Africa at the height of the typhoid epidemic that developed at every British military encampment. Doyle had been vaccinated against typhoid before leaving England and was critical of allowing typhoid vaccination to be voluntary for soldiers. In Africa, he was appalled at the level of disease. During the three months he was there, he reported that there were 5,000 cases of typhoid and 1,000 deaths among soldiers and many more among civilians. Over the entire course of the war, about 58,000 soldiers developed typhoid and 9,000 died. Despite the death toll, mandatory military vaccination in Britain was not reinstated until after World War I (1914–1918).

VACCINE ACCEPTANCE IN THE UNITED STATES

At the start of the 19th century, scientists did not understand that microorganisms caused contagious diseases. This led to many theories about infection, including the ideas that diseases were caused by an act of God, brought on by environmental factors, or occurred because of imbalances in the humors (fluids) in the body. Nevertheless, vaccination was better received in the United States than in England.

Smallpox vaccine was introduced to America by a British physician who sent Benjamin Waterhouse (1745–1846), a professor at Harvard University in Massachusetts, a sample soon after the vaccine became available. In 1800, Waterhouse, a supporter of vaccination, sent some vaccine to Vice President Thomas Jefferson (1743–1826). Jefferson was intensely interested in the possibilities of vaccination. He reportedly vaccinated about 200 neighbors and members of his household and during his presidency (1801–1809) created the National Vaccine Institute. His presidential successor, James Madison (1751–1836), signed the Vaccine Act of 1813. The Act was repealed nine years later. After that, there was little organized opposition to vaccination for 30 years. Any regulation of vaccination became the responsibility of individual states.

AMERICAN VACCINE RESISTANCE GROWS

In 1852, Massachusetts became the first state to provide free public education to all children and to make school attendance compulsory. Children from all backgrounds now shared crowded classrooms, making schools the perfect setting for the spread of contagious diseases. Public health officials recognized the danger. A single case of smallpox in one classroom could spread the disease throughout an entire town. Consequently, in 1855, Massachusetts began requiring proof of smallpox vaccination for public school attendance. Parents opposed to vaccination could still send their children to private school or have them tutored at home, and there were provisions for medical exemptions from the law. Other states gradually followed Massachusetts in linking vaccinations to school attendance. Today, all 50 states require either proof of certain vaccinations or proof of a medical, religious, or personal belief exemption for children to attend public schools and often private schools and daycare centers. All states allow medical exemptions, but availability of religious and personal belief exemptions vary by state.

Anti-vaccination sentiment grew as more states passed and enforced mandatory vaccination laws, but challenges to vaccination were less organized than in Britain because there were no national vaccine laws, and state laws and enforcement varied widely. The movement got a boost when British anti-vaccination activist William Tebb (1830–1919) visited New York in 1879 and helped to establish the Anti-Vaccination Society of America. This was followed by the establishment of the New England

Anti-Compulsory Vaccination League in 1882 and the Anti-Vaccination League of New York City in 1885. Anti-vaccination books and pamphlets circulated widely. Tebb's *Vaccines and Leprosy,* for example, blamed the increase in leprosy on smallpox vaccination.

Jacobson v. Massachusetts

Massachusetts was the first state to make vaccination against smallpox a condition for children to attend public school. The law also allowed public health officials to require vaccination of all individuals of any age if an outbreak of smallpox occurred. Individuals who refused could be fined.

These laws were tested when there was an outbreak of smallpox in Cambridge, Massachusetts, in 1902. Pastor Henning Jacobson, a Cambridge resident, claimed to have been vaccinated in his native Sweden and said the procedure had caused him lifelong pain and suffering. He refused vaccination, but he also refused to pay the fine. Instead, he went to court. He lost but appealed the case. *Jacobson v. Massachusetts* went all the way to the U.S. Supreme Court. In 1905, Jacobson lost the Supreme Court appeal by a 7–2 vote. This case established a precedent for mandatory vaccination. A discussion of the case and its continuing implications is found in Chapter 12.

THE MODERN VACCINE DEBATE

For the first 75 years of the 20th century, there were individual outcries against vaccination, but organized resistance was low. In Britain, George Bernard Shaw (1856–1950), Irish playwright and Nobel Prize winner, carried on a crusade against vaccination in letters to the *British Medical Journal* and the *Irish Times*. He considered vaccination "a particularly filthy piece of witchcraft" and "nothing short of murder." He labeled the *British Medical Journal* "bigotedly vaccinist" (Shaw, 1901).

In the United States, a case was brought against the city of San Antonio in 1919 that again tested the legality of mandatory vaccinations in school children. The Supreme Court in 1922 refuse to hear the case, and a lower court ruling in favor of the city's laws requiring vaccination was upheld (see Chapter 12).

During the 1960s, new vaccines for children including those against measles, mumps, and rubella were introduced. With these new vaccines came an increase in organized anti-vaccination activity. Once again, the movement began in England where, in 1974, Rosemary Fox founded the

Association of Parents of Vaccine Damaged Children. Fox documented her daughter's experience in the book *Helen's Story.*

In 1962, Helen Fox had been given inactivated polio vaccine at the age of eight months. The day after the shot, she developed projectile vomiting that was treated with medication. Then, four months later, Helen began having seizures and developmental delays. When she was 11 years old, she was assessed as having a mental age of a 3-year-old. At that point, her mother, Rosemary, decided that the polio vaccine given to her when she was eight months old had damaged her.

Fox solicited information from other parents who believed their children had been damaged by any vaccine, not just polio vaccine. Using this information, she enlisted Member of Parliament Jack Ashley, later to become Lord Ashley of Stoke, to push for government financial compensation for vaccine damages. Twenty-seven years later, even though legal liability for vaccine damage had not been established, the British government made payments to Fox and other parents who had joined the Association of Parents of Vaccine Damaged Children.

VACCINE RESISTANCE APPEARS IN AMERICA

Just as in the early years of smallpox vaccination, concern about vaccine safety crossed the Atlantic from Britain and found a receptive home in the United States. On April 19, 1982, the NBC affiliate WRC-TV in Washington, D.C., broadcast an hour-long documentary called *DPT: Vaccine Roulette.* The program's writer and host, Lea Thompson, head of WRC's consumer unit, interviewed parents who asserted that their children had been harmed by the pertussis component of the diphtheria, pertussis, and tetanus (DPT) shot. These parents described previously normal children who experienced seizures, developmental regression, and permanent mental and physical disabilities in the weeks and months following vaccination. The program resonated with the public and was rebroadcast several times. Thompson claimed that more than 2,000 people called the station after seeing the program. Many reported that they believed their child, like children profiled in the broadcast, had been harmed by the DPT vaccine.

DPT: Vaccine Roulette was controversial. After the broadcast, the American Academy of Pediatrics called the program "unfortunate and dangerous" (Hilts, 1982) and expressed concern that resistance to vaccinating with DPT would lead to a pertussis outbreak. This had already occurred in Japan when a scare about pertussis vaccine caused a drop in coverage from 80 percent in 1974 to 10 percent in 1976, followed by an outbreak of 13,000 pertussis cases and 41 deaths three years later. Other physicians criticized the program for showing 11 minutes of footage of supposedly vaccine-damaged children and their families and less than 2 minutes of a child suffering from whooping cough. They also challenged the accuracy of some of Thompson's facts, including a statistic that 1 of every 700 children was damaged by DPT vaccination. Vaccine scientists accepted that complications could occur from the pertussis component of DPT, but they claimed the rate of serious injury was only 1 in 100,000, or about 50 cases per year in the United States.

Barbara Loe Fisher was one of the parents who saw *DPT: Vaccine Roulette* and believed it explained why her healthy two-and-a half-year-old son had regressed physically, mentally, and emotionally not long after his fourth DPT shot. She claimed the shot had caused encephalopathy (brain inflammation) that left him with attention deficit disorder and autism.

Fisher, along with several other parents who felt their children also had been damaged by DPT, formed the organization Dissatisfied Parents Together. Creation of this organization is generally accepted as the start of the modern anti-vaccination movement in the United States. The organization was politically active and was instrumental in the federal government taking more responsibility for vaccine injuries through the National Vaccine Injury Compensation Program (see Chapter 4).

Dissatisfied Parents Together changed its name to the National Vaccine Information Center (NVIC) and expanded its vaccine resistance to other vaccines, especially the measles, mumps, and rubella (MMR) combination vaccine. Barbara Loe Fisher and NVIC's continuing role in the vaccine controversy is discussed in more detail in Chapter 10.

VACCINE RESISTANCE SPREADS

In the late 1990s, multiple trends came together to accelerate the anti-vaccination movement.

- The chickenpox, hepatitis A, and rotavirus vaccines were licensed. Many parents perceived these vaccine-preventable diseases as minor and became increasingly skeptical about profit motives of big pharmaceutical companies pushing use of these new vaccines.
- People became more concerned about chemicals in processed foods and in the environment. Demand for organic or "natural" products increased.
- The passage of the 1994 Dietary Supplement Health and Education Act required the U.S. Food and Drug Administration (FDA) to

regulate nutritional supplements (vitamins, minerals, and herbs) as foods rather than applying more stringent regulations used to verify the safety of pharmaceutical drugs. Demand for nutritional and herbal remedies exploded among consumers who viewed them as safer and more natural replacements for traditional drugs.

- Alternative medicine practices such as functional medicine, naturopathic medicine, holistic healing, nutritional medicine, chiropractic medicine, herbal treatments, traditional Chinese medicine, and Ayurvedic medicine (traditional Indian medicine) became more visible and more accepted.

- Home computers became affordable, making the Internet available to many more people. Newsgroups developed around specific topics, allowing people to share their experiences with like-minded people. Open Diary, a way for people to record their daily lives on the web, began in 1998, and blogs soon followed. Public blogs and personal websites created an uncensored platform for user-generated content, allowing anti-vaccinationists to connect and promote their views.

These forces gathered steam through the 1990s, and then came the spark that lit the fuse that spread the anti-vaccination movement across much of the world. And that spark came from a member of the traditional medical community.

In 1998, Andrew Wakefield (1957–), a physician and gastroenterology researcher at the Royal Free Hospital in London, called a press conference to announce that research done by him and 12 colleagues showed that the MMR vaccine was associated with the development of autism. He particularly identified the measles component of the vaccine as the problematic element. British media treated this announcement as credible and newsworthy because the research was published in the reputable, peer-reviewed British journal, *The Lancet.* Soon parents began rejecting MMR vaccination for their children. The story spread across Europe, to Australia, Japan, and the United States, where it was publicized by Barbara Loe Fisher and the NVIC.

In reality, the published research *did not* support Wakefield's conclusion. Ten of his research colleagues immediately rejected his statements. The paper was later retracted (declared invalid), and Wakefield lost his license to practice medicine because of conflicts of interest and unethical behavior surrounding this research. Nevertheless, by the time the scientific community had studied and rejected the MMR–autism connection, Wakefield's theory had been publicized worldwide. More details of the controversy can be found in Chapter 10.

MORE FUEL FOR VACCINE SKEPTICS

In the United States, two other events added to the vaccine debate. The first occurred when the public became aware that some vaccines contained a preservative called thimerosal that is about 50 percent mercury by weight. Thimerosal had been used without controversy to prevent the growth of bacteria and fungi in drugs since the 1930s. It came to the attention of the public only when the FDA published a review of foods and drugs containing mercury. In 1999, the FDA, with the support of the National Institutes of Health, the Centers for Disease Control and Prevention (CDC), the American Academy of Pediatrics, and the American Academy of Family Physicians, sent a letter to vaccine manufacturers requesting that they remove thimerosal from vaccines. Then the FDA muddied the situation by claiming that there was no evidence that thimerosal caused harm. People naturally questioned why, if thimerosal caused no harm, had the FDA asked that it be taken out of vaccines.

Mercury in some forms, although not in the form found in thimerosal, is a known neurotoxin. In the United States, the thimerosal issue quickly became conflated with Andrew Wakefield's claim that MMR vaccine caused autism. Soon vaccine skeptics were claiming that MMR vaccine caused autism because it contained thimerosal. Congressional hearings were held on this issue and were covered widely by the press (see Chapter 10). By 2001, manufacturers no longer added thimerosal to vaccines in the United States for children under age six years except for influenza vaccine.

Anti-vaccinationists were not satisfied. They continued to demanded proof that vaccines did not cause autism and developmental delays. In 2005, journalist David Kirby (1960–) published *Evidence of Harm—Mercury in Vaccines and the Autism Epidemic: A Medical Controversy.* The book kept the vaccine-autism debate in the public eye. It claimed that because scientists were not able to prove definitively that MMR *did not* cause autism or other harm, it remained possible that it did. This illogical argument requiring proof of a negative event energized anti-vaccinationists who then claimed that MMR vaccination posed an unnecessary risk.

About the same time, a second incident aroused consumer concern about vaccine safety. In 1999, RotaShield, a vaccine against rotavirus, an organism that causes severe and sometimes fatal diarrhea and dehydration in infants, was voluntarily withdrawn from the market. Postlicensing surveillance data suggested that in children under one year of age, RotaShield slightly increased the chance of intussusception, a rare condition in which one part of the bowel folds in on itself, causing a life-threatening blockage.

Anti-vaccination parents claimed that the withdrawal of RotaShield meant that "big pharma" was pushing harmful vaccines on innocent children and hiding data that showed they caused damage in the name of profits.

GREEN OUR VACCINES

Despite the discrediting of Wakefield's work by reputable scientists and the fact that thimerosal was no longer used in vaccines, the anti-vaccination movement continued to gain increased visibility through the 2000s. One reason was the involvement of celebrity anti-vaccinationists who could command attention from the media. Jenny McCarthy, a former *Playboy* Playmate of the Year, actress, and author, along with her then boyfriend, actor Jim Carrey, were two of the most visible celebrity anti-vaccinationists. McCarthy's son, Evan, was diagnosed with autism in 2005. After educating herself at what McCarthy called the University of Google, she claimed her "mommy instinct" told her that vaccines had caused her son's medical problems. She set out to publicize her experience in a book and with appearances in 2007 on *The Oprah Winfrey Show, Larry King Live,* and *Good Morning America.* On these programs, seen by millions of parents, she blamed vaccines for her son's autism and praised Andrew Wakefield's work.

McCarthy also joined forces with Generation Rescue, an organization that blamed combination vaccines for autism. Together McCarthy and Generation Rescue conducted a highly visible media campaign against vaccination. Other organizations such as Autism Speaks, SafeMinds, and Talk About Curing Autism joined McCarthy in promoting the explanation that vaccines and other environmental factors cause autism. (Autism Speaks and TACA have since backed away from this position.)

In June 2008, McCarthy and Carrey led a Green Our Vaccines rally in Washington, D.C., to protest vaccine additives, combination vaccines, and the CDC-recommended vaccination schedule. The celebrity component guaranteed media coverage. One of the speakers was Robert Kennedy, Jr., environmental activist and anti-vaccinationist. McCarthy and Generation Rescue also established the AutismOne conference where vaccine opponents promoted their views.

CHANGING TACTICS

Meanwhile, no reputable scientific study found any connection between vaccines and autism. As the negative evidence piled up (often rejected by anti-vaccinationists as a lack of evidence), anti-vaccine organizations began to change their tactics. Today, vaccine-skeptic organizations such as the NVIC in the United States and the Australian Vaccination-Skeptics Network claim they are not "anti-vaccine" but "pro safe vaccine."

Despite the wording change, these organizations continue to insist that the safety of vaccines has not been adequately proven, that combination vaccines cause antigen overload, and that government-recommended vaccination schedules include unnecessary vaccines and require too many vaccines at too young an age. Although these organizations present their position as pro safe vaccines, they strongly support a parent's right to reject some or all vaccinations or to have vaccines administered on an alternative schedule (see Chapter 11). Some of the more extreme organizations and anti-vaccination websites continue to promote the theory that there is a conspiracy between the government and pharmaceutical companies to hide data that show vaccines are toxic (see Chapter 13).

Vaccine resistance has existed for as long as the procedure has been used and is likely to continue as new vaccines are developed. Reasons for vaccine skepticism are varied and include belief that vaccines are ineffective, faith-based objections, belief that vaccines cause harm, concern that mandatory vaccination violates personal liberty, and, in extreme cases, belief that vaccines are a part of a conspiracy between pharmaceutical companies and the government. The media and the internet have played a major role in modern times in spreading or maintaining these objections. Scientific research showing the safety, effectiveness, and benefits of vaccination has done little to change the minds of anti-vaccinationists who continue to find reasons to label this research as inadequate, incomplete, or unreliable.

PART II

Issues and Controversies

CHAPTER 7

Why Vaccines Are Controversial

Attitudes toward vaccines range from complete acceptance to complete rejection. Most people accept vaccinations as a routine life-saving preventative measure. Nevertheless, a substantial number of people question their safety and utility. That number is increasing, especially in developed countries. Anti-vaccinationists can be divided into two main groups. Vaccination refusers oppose all vaccinations. This group comprises between 2 percent and 4 percent of the parents in many developed countries. Vaccine skeptics oppose some vaccinations but accept others and/or reject the government-recommended schedule of vaccinations. Forty percent of French parents and about 30 percent of parents in the United States and Great Britain fall into this category. Vaccine skeptics also make up a substantial percentage of parents in countries as diverse as Romania, Italy, Australia, and Japan.

Although they have opposing views of vaccines, the acceptors, rejectors, and vaccine skeptics all believe that they are doing what is best for their children. So how did concerned adults arrive at such different conclusions about the value of vaccination? Attitudes appear to be influenced by the individual's interpretation of statistical information, unconscious psychological factors, exposure to vaccine narratives, and personal experience.

EVALUATING RISK

Risk assessment is the process of determining the probability of a negative event occurring in a defined population based on historical data. It is possible to quite accurately determine what will happen to a large group of people based on what has happened in the past, but risk assessment can never predict what will happen to any single individual in the group. For example, actuarial tables for life insurance in the United States are based on the age at which millions of Americans have died. They quite accurately determine the life expectancy of the hypothetical average person, but they say nothing about individual life expectancy. Some people will die before age 50 and others live to be 100—and there is no way to predict who will draw the long-life straw and whose life will end prematurely.

The same situation occurs with risk assessment of a vaccine. The statistical risk of an adverse effect (i.e., a reaction provably caused by the vaccine) is calculated by comparing the number of doses of vaccine administered to the number of adverse effects occurring in a defined period after vaccination. Adverse effects are categorized as mild (e.g., transient soreness at the injection site, low to moderate fever), moderate (e.g., jerking, staring, fever over 105°F [40.5°C]), or serious (e.g., allergic reaction, long-term seizures, brain damage). Depending on the vaccine, mild adverse effects such as soreness at the injection site are common, often occurring in 15–20 percent of those vaccinated, while serious adverse effects occur at the rate of less than 1–2 per million doses. Calculation of adverse effects is a reasonably accurate representation of risk from vaccination, but like lifetime actuarial tables, it says nothing about whether a vaccine will cause an undesirable reaction in any specific individual.

Risk of contracting a disease is calculated by comparing the number of cases of the disease to the size of a population. Again, risk calculation gives a prediction across an entire population but says nothing about any single individual. In addition, calculation of the risk of contracting a vaccine-preventable disease is complicated by other factors. Some vaccine-preventable diseases are far more likely to have serious complications in certain age groups. For example, children under age two are more susceptible to rotavirus and *Haemophilus influenzae* type b (Hib) infection and are more likely to develop serious or life-threatening diarrhea (rotavirus) or bacterial meningitis (Hib) than older children. On the other hand, chickenpox and measles are more serious diseases in adults than in children, and rubella (German measles) is a mild disease, but in pregnant women can cause life-altering birth defects in a developing fetus.

When disease risk is calculated across an entire population and vaccine adverse effects are calculated only for vaccinated children, it becomes difficult for parents to make an accurate, reasoned evaluation of risk. Instead, parents tend to make decisions based on stories they have heard about vaccines, attitudes of other parents in their peer group, and their own gut feelings about the reliability of the medical establishment and pharmaceutical industry.

The number of vaccinated individuals in the local community also complicates determining the risk of contracting a disease compared to the risk associated with immunization against it. Herd immunity occurs when enough people are vaccinated against a disease to limit its ability to spread. The percentage of coverage to establish herd immunity varies with the contagiousness of the disease. For example, about 94 percent of the community must be vaccinated against measles or pertussis (whooping cough) to establish effective herd immunity. The percentage for most other vaccine-preventable diseases is in the 85–90 percent range. However, in some communities with active anti-vaccination advocates, 25–30 percent of kindergarten children are unvaccinated or incompletely vaccinated. This percentage is inadequate to establish herd immunity, so children in low vaccine-coverage communities are at higher risk of contracting a vaccine-preventable disease.

Lifestyle is another factor influencing risk. Families who travel abroad frequently or have visitors coming from developing countries or areas where vaccine-preventable diseases are common are more likely to be exposed to these diseases. In addition, children who have been fully vaccinated and show no symptoms of illness can carry a vaccine-preventable infection home from a contagious child at school or daycare. Siblings who may be too young to be vaccinated or whose vaccinations have been delayed are then put at risk for becoming ill.

How We Perceive Risk

For a parent in the developed world with little or no firsthand experience with most vaccine-preventable diseases, deciding whether to vaccinate is more complicated than comparing statistics. Behavioral scientists who study response to risk have found multiple biases influence the way people perceive and evaluate potentially harmful events.

- Confirmation bias: Behavioral research shows that people put more trust in information that confirms what they already believe than in information that challenges their belief system. Parents with anti-vaccinationist leanings are more likely to believe and act on information that shows vaccines are harmful, even when the reported studies have not been peer-reviewed or have been performed by discredited individuals and are outweighed by dozens of quality studies that have found the opposite to be true. Vaccine acceptors are more likely to believe studies that show vaccines protect against disease. These biases tend to lead to a hardening of attitudes toward vaccination on both sides of the debate.

- Omission bias: Individuals are more likely to regret events that occur in response to an action they have taken rather than events that occur from a failure to act. Because of this bias, parents are more likely to feel they are at fault if their child has an adverse reaction to a vaccine, even a mild or moderate one, than they are if their child later contracts a vaccine-preventable disease. No one wants to feel guilty about a decision, so the default position is often to do nothing rather than take the risk of giving a healthy child a vaccine that might cause a negative response.

- Availability bias: Availability bias arises from access to information, whether true or false. There is a proven tendency to let the first story or example that comes to mind influence a decision. A health care worker or parent who knows someone who has experienced a vaccine-preventable disease is most likely to think of this person and their illness when vaccines are mentioned. On the other hand, the false narrative that certain vaccines cause autism has been around for decades. Most parents have heard stories about autism, know someone with an autistic child, or have seen vaccine-skeptic websites that publish heartbreaking stories of parents who insist that their child's autism was caused by a vaccine because symptoms developed soon after an inoculation. Although the link between autism and vaccination has been discredited by dozens of high-quality studies, these studies do not get the same press coverage or have the same emotional impact as first-person accounts of vaccine tragedies. Stories of vaccine damage may come quickly to mind, stimulating fear that one's own children could be harmed and in that way influence the decision to vaccinate.

- Temporal bias: Humans are far better at recognizing and responding to events that can cause damage in the immediate future than they are to threats where damage is delayed or uncertain. For example, people caught in a thunderstorm perceive a real, although very small, risk of being struck by lightning. They respond by seeking safe shelter. These same people, however, may smoke cigarettes for years, even though they know that smoking can cause lung cancer. The statistical risk of a smoker developing lung cancer is far greater than the statistical risk of being struck by lightning. Nevertheless, the perceived risk of being struck by lightning in the present motivates a change in behavior while the risk of developing lung cancer in the future does not. In terms of vaccination, the chance of an adverse reaction from a vaccine is immediate, making the risk seem larger, while the risk of contracting the disease that the vaccine protects against appears smaller because it may happen far in the future or not at all. This disconnect can influence the decision whether to delay or to decline vaccination.

• Optimism bias: Behavioral scientists tell us that most people are naturally optimistic. Optimists believe that bad things may happen to other people but will never happen to them. This kind of thinking keeps casinos in business. Gamblers know that the house always wins, but each gambler believes that even though the other guy may lose money, he will walk away a winner. Natural optimism adds to the difficulty of accurately assessing risk. Optimist parents understand that some unvaccinated children may become ill or even die from vaccine-preventable diseases, but they discount the idea that their child will be the one who gets sick. When optimism is factored into the risk equation, parents may ask why they should accept *any* level of risk from vaccinating.

Most people accept vaccination as a health benefit; however, about one-third of parents in developed countries either reject some vaccines or choose to alter the government-recommended vaccination schedule. These decisions are often based on parental perception of the risk of vaccinating versus the risk of developing a vaccine-preventable disease combined with distrust of the medical establishment's interpretation of these risks.

Risk can be determined accurately for large populations, but this risk determination gives little information about the fate of any particular individual in the group. Difficulty in analyzing risk along with emotional factors complicates some parents' decision on whether to vaccinate. These emotional factors include confirmation bias, omission bias, availability bias, temporal bias, and optimism bias. Both pro-vaccinationists and anti-vaccinationists believe their choices are in the best interest of their children. This has led to the hardening of positions on both sides.

The following chapters look in detail at some common issues that arise in the vaccine debate. The background of each issue is outlined, followed by the vaccine-skeptic view and the medical establishment view on the controversy. When reading these contradictory viewpoints, keep in mind the reliability of the source of information, whether the information is presented in context, and the biases that affect the interpretation of the information.

CHAPTER 8

Do Vaccines Prevent Disease?

As many as 4 percent of Americans are complete vaccine rejectors. These anti-vaccinationists give a variety of reasons for refusing all immunizations including their belief that vaccines simply do not work. This attitude baffles and frustrates the medical establishment. It believes it has provided overwhelming reliable data that show vaccines are effective in reducing contagious diseases. However, the belief that vaccines are useless has considerable history. In America, this idea took root in the late 1800s and persists to this day.

BACKGROUND

At the end of the 19th century, medical education in the United States was quite different from medical education today. Initially, medical schools were associated with universities, but by the middle of the 18th century, freestanding medical institutes were common in both cities and small towns. Virtually any man (women usually were barred) could buy himself a seat at one of these independent institutions. Professors were paid out of student fees, so the schools had financial incentive to enroll as many students as possible.

Teaching took place in large lecture halls with little or no hands-on training. Courses were not graded, even at university-associated medical schools such as Harvard. There were no educational prerequisites for enrollment until 1898, when Johns Hopkins University began requiring people attending its medical school to first earn a bachelor's degree. Harvard followed suit a few years later, but at the start of the 20th century, practically any man willing to pay the fees could call himself a medical doctor.

Given the poor state of medical education, many people were afraid, or at least skeptical, of doctors. Even well-intentioned physicians prescribed treatments such as bloodletting, arsenic, and mercury that did more harm than good. Traditional medicine competed with folk remedies, homeopathy, hydrotherapy, faith healing, and all types of unregulated patent medicines, some of which were useless and some of which were lethal. Patients had few ways to distinguish helpful treatments from frauds.

This was the health care situation in 1897 when Daniel David Palmer (1845–1913) established the first School of Chiropractic Medicine in Davenport, Iowa. Palmer rejected the germ theory of disease which states that pathogens entering the body are the cause of infectious illness. Instead, he taught that illness was caused by misalignment of the joints and could be cured by joint manipulation. Because he rejected the germ theory on which vaccination is based, Palmer had no use for vaccines. He called vaccination "a medical delusion" and vaccines "filthy animal poison" (Gleberzon, 2013). His son, Bartlett Joshua Palmer (1882–1961), went further, stating "chiropractors have found in every disease that is supposed to be contagious a cause in the spine . . . There is no contagious disease . . . There is no infection . . . The idea of poisoning healthy people with vaccine . . . is irrational" (Gleberzon, 2013).

Homeopaths also had no use for vaccines. George Winterburn (b. 1845), a New York homeopath, wrote *The Value of Vaccination,* in which he claimed that vaccination had no scientific basis and was a worthless fad. Instead, homeopathic practitioners offered their own inoffensive but ineffective alternatives to vaccines. Faith healers preached that the body was perfect as it was. God, they claimed, would heal illness if various faith rituals were performed. For them, vaccination was both unnatural and unnecessary. All these groups encouraged vaccine refusal, but since only a few states had rigorous compulsory vaccination laws, there was little large-scale organized resistance.

MODERN ANTI-VACCINATIONIST VIEWS

Anti-vaccinationists who believe vaccines do not work use arguments similar to those from one hundred years ago. Today, the Palmers' rejection of the germ theory and of vaccines continues to be supported by some segments of the chiropractic community. Chiropractor Brad Case, owner of the now-closed Holistic Healing Center in Prunedale, California, is a germ theory denialist. Case subscribes to a new germ theory that he calls the theory of pleomorphism. He bases his theory on the assertions of Antoine Béchamp (1816–1908), a 19th-century French doctor. Béchamp claimed that he found tiny mobile granules within cells that are the basis for life. He called these granules microzymas. According to the theory of pleomorphism, "Under toxic conditions, microzymas would change into what we think of as disease-causing microorganisms, i.e. viruses, bacteria, fungi, and parasites" (Case, 2010, 152). This theory postulates that certain things we eat, inhale, think, and feel assault the body. When the body is attacked, healthy microzymas change into disease-causing pathogens. In other words, disease comes from within us, not from outside pathogens.

Another anti-vaccination website makes a similar argument from Dr. Henry Bieler (1893–1975), author of *Food Is Your Best Medicine.* Bieler says, "The primary cause of disease is not germs. Rather, I believe disease is caused by a toxemia which results in cellular impairment and breakdown" (International Foundation for Nutrition and Health, n.d.). The corollary of both these beliefs is that if we eat correctly, avoid toxins, and maintain the proper emotional state, we will remain healthy; therefore, vaccination is both unnecessary and harmful.

Other anti-vaccinationists suggest that the decrease in contagious diseases has occurred independent of vaccination. Sherri Tenpenny, an American anti-vaccine osteopathic doctor, writes "Public health officials attribute low infection rates to mandatory vaccination policies rather than giving credit to improved personal hygiene and modern conveniences such as indoor plumbing . . . Vaccines provide false security about protection" (Merino, 2015, 57).

VaxTruth, another anti-vaccination website, states that modern medicine is not responsible for and has played little part in substantially improved life expectancy and survival from disease in Western economies. The website claims that the main advances in combating disease over 200 years have been better food and clean drinking water. It makes this claim despite a graph on its own website that shows a dramatic drop in measles cases soon after the vaccine came into widespread use. Vaccine rejectors also claim that vaccines do not work because as many or more vaccinated than unvaccinated people get sick during a disease outbreak (see Table 8.1).

MAINSTREAM MEDICAL VIEWS

Vaccines work, and vaccination saves lives and prevents disability. That is the position of virtually every traditional medical organization, including the U.S. Centers for Disease Control and Prevention, the U.S. Institute of Medicine, the World Health Organization, and virtually all national medical accrediting organizations. Some vaccines are more effective than

others. Some provide longer protection than others, but overall, vaccination is an effective way to reduce infectious disease, and that is because
the germ theory—the idea that pathogens enter the body and cause infectious diseases—is correct. This theory is supported by more than 150 years
of worldwide scientific research, and no alternative theory adequately
explains disease transmission.

Access to clean water, better sewage treatment, improved food sanitation, better nutrition, advances in medical treatment, and increased access
to health care have contributed to the decline of many contagious diseases.
Nevertheless, if these changes were the only reason vaccine-preventable
diseases have decreased, one would expect a simultaneous and gradual
reduction in many diseases over the same time period. Instead, statistics
show that reductions in various vaccine-preventable diseases have occurred
independently of each other, and each disease has shown a sudden steep
decline shortly after a vaccine against it became widely available.

Chickenpox provides a good example. Before the chickenpox (varicella) vaccine was licensed in 1995, about four million cases of chickenpox occurred in the United States each year. By 2004, there were about
600,000 cases, or 85 percent fewer than before widespread vaccination.
Ten years later, in 2015, the number had dropped further to about 151,000
cases. If only improved living conditions were responsible, the number
of cases would have declined slowly and gradually as living conditions
improved rather than taking a sudden dip. The same sudden decrease can
be seen, for example, after introduction of measles and rotavirus vaccines.

Vaccines are extremely effective, but very occasionally vaccinated individuals do become ill with a disease they have been vaccinated against.
There are several reasons for this. In diseases with long incubation times
(e.g., measles), a person may be infected before vaccination but not show
symptoms until after receiving the vaccine. In other cases, the individual's
immune system may not respond adequately to the vaccine because of an
undetected immune system deficiency. This is uncommon. The most likely
cause for apparent vaccine failure is because the individual was incompletely vaccinated and/or has skipped the needed booster shots to maintain
immunity.

Despite the demonstrated effectiveness of immunization, anti-
vaccinationists claim that during outbreaks of a vaccine-preventable disease, as many or more vaccinated people contract the disease as those
people who are not vaccinated. This statement, although numerically
true, is highly misleading. An accurate statement is that the *percentage*
of vaccinated individuals who get sick in a disease outbreak is much
lower than the *percentage* of unvaccinated individuals.

Table 8.1 Comparison of Absolute Number and Percentage of People Contracting a Disease after Vaccination with a 98% Effective Vaccine

Total population	500		
Total vaccinated	490		
Number who develop immunity and stay healthy	480	Percentage who stay healthy	98
Number vaccinated but not immune who get sick	10	Percentage who get sick	2
Number not vaccinated and *not* immune who get sick	10	Percentage who get sick	100

Source: College of Physicians of Philadelphia https://www.historyofvaccines.org.

The College of Physicians of Philadelphia provides this example. A group of 500 people are exposed to a disease. Ten are not vaccinated and 490 are vaccinated with a vaccine that is 98 percent effective. This results in a population of 480 people (98%) who develop immunity, 10 (2%) who remain vulnerable after vaccination for one of the reasons listed earlier, and 10 (100%) vulnerable unvaccinated individuals.

If all the vulnerable individuals get sick when exposed to the disease, then 10 vaccinated and 10 unvaccinated individuals will contract the disease. However, as indicated in Table 8.1, although the absolute numbers are the same, only 2 percent of vaccinated people get sick, while 100 percent of unvaccinated people get sick. The odds clearly favor the vaccinated people staying healthy, showing that vaccination does work.

CHAPTER 9

Are Vaccines Adequately Tested for Safety?

Vaccine development and production in the United States are regulated by the federal government. As discussed in Chapter 4, the backbone of this regulation is the 1902 Biologics Control Act that sets standards for the production of antitoxins, serums, and vaccines and the 1906 Pure Food, Drug, and Cosmetic Act that oversees drug safety. Both these Acts have been amended many times to improve drug safety and to keep up with advances in medical technology. Nevertheless, anti-vaccinationists and the mainstream medical establishment have a fundamental disagreement over whether the testing of vaccines required by these Acts and their amendments is adequate to assure their safety.

BACKGROUND

The safety of vaccines is regulated by national and international law in all developed countries. In the United States, responsibility is assigned to the Center for Biologics Evaluation and Research within the Food and Drug Administration. Vaccine safety is regulated in Canada by the Biologics and Genetic Therapies Directorate, in Australia by the Therapeutic Goods Administration, and in the European Union by the European Medicines Agency. The World Health Organization (WHO) has its own set of vaccine safety standards that many other countries have adopted. The goal of these regulations is twofold: to assure vaccines are safe and effective before they are licensed for public use and to assure their continued purity throughout the manufacturing process.

In the United States, the results of pre- and postlicensure studies are evaluated by the government-mandated Advisory Committee on Immunization Practices (ACIP), which then makes recommendations on their use. The voting committee consists of 14 medical professionals and 1 consumer representative. They are aided by 30 nonvoting vaccine experts who represent organizations involved in immunization programs such as the Global Action Vaccine Plan. Although ACIP recommendations are not binding, they form the basis of the vaccine schedule recommended by the Centers for Disease Control and Prevention (CDC). Most physicians follow this schedule.

WHO recommendations are developed by the Strategic Advisory Group of Experts (SAGE) on Immunization. These recommendations are the basis for the WHO's Global Vaccine Action Plan that aims to strengthen and extend coverage of routine vaccinations worldwide. SAGE recommendations may differ from CDC recommendations based on the needs and limitations of various national immunization programs and the prevalence of disease in different parts of the world. The goal of both organizations is to use objective data to maximize public health benefits of vaccination while minimizing health risks to individuals.

ANTI-VACCINATIONIST VIEWS ON SAFETY

"We're not an anti-vaccine movement . . . We're pro-safe vaccine," celebrity Jenny McCarthy, spokesperson for the anti-vaccination organization Generation Rescue, told the television program *Frontline* (Public Broadcasting System, 2015). Sherry Tenpenny, an anti-vaccinationist osteopath, sums up this argument when she states "vaccines have never been proven safe by the gold standard of medical research: The double-blind, placebo-controlled investigation" (Merino, 2015, 54).

A double-blind placebo-controlled study is one in which two groups of participants matched for age and health status are injected either with a vaccine or with a harmless substance such as a saline (mild salt water). Neither the health care workers running the study nor the participants know whether they are getting the vaccine or the placebo. The response of participants is tested and evaluated, and the results of the two groups are compared statistically to determine the effectiveness of the vaccine and the rate of side effects occurring in each group.

Aluminum in Vaccines

The active part of any vaccine is the antigen that stimulates an immune system response leading to the development of memory cells (see Chapter 2), but vaccines contain other components that are dissolved in a suspending fluid. Depending on the vaccine, the suspending fluid may contain stabilizers to shield against temperature changes (vaccines are highly temperature-sensitive), preservatives or antibiotics to prevent contamination, adjuvants to boost antigen performance, and production residues, which are miniscule amounts of materials remaining after growing and processing the antigen (see Chapter 3 for details on vaccine components).

For many years, the preservative thimerosal, a chemical that can be broken down into one form of mercury, was a source of safety concerns surrounding vaccines (see Chapter 10). Thimerosal was removed from most vaccines beginning in 2001, and a thimerosal-free version of all childhood vaccines is now available in the United States. Since thimerosal is no longer added to vaccines, safety challenges have shifted to adjuvant compounds that contain aluminum, which is used to boost effectiveness of the antigen. Aluminum serves as an adjuvant in vaccines against hepatitis A, hepatitis B, diphtheria-tetanus-pertussis (DTaP), *Haemophilus influenzae* type b (Hib), human papillomavirus (HPV), and pneumococcus.

According to anti-vaccinationists, the safety of aluminum in vaccines has been inadequately studied and therefore is potentially dangerous. Anti-vaccination activist Jenny McCarthy is on record as saying that now that thimerosal has been eliminated from childhood vaccines, "Aluminum is the other devil, so to speak. It's a heavy metal that's in vaccines much more, I believe, than mercury ever was" (Public Broadcasting System, 2015). After California governor Jerry Brown signed a mandatory state vaccination law in 2015, anti-vaccine actor Jim Carrey told *Time* magazine "California Gov says yes to poisoning more children with mercury and aluminium in manditory [*sic*] vaccines. This corporate fascist must be stopped" (Kluger, 2015).

The Vaccine Injury Compensation Program

Anti-vaccinationists point to the existence of the Vaccine Injury Compensation Program (VICP), a government program that compensates individuals provably damaged by a vaccine, as the government's admission that vaccines are not adequately safe. The VICP operates outside the civil court system and provides a faster way for vaccine-injured individuals to receive compensation than bringing a liability case in civil court.

For a damaged individual to receive compensation, the vaccine must be on the CDC list of recommended vaccines for routine administration to children. Adult vaccines and vaccines given to special populations such as travelers or the military are not covered by the program. In addition, the type of damage should be listed in the official Vaccine Injury Table (VIT) and occur within a designated time frame.

Disabilities and injuries caused by adulterants or contaminants in a vaccine are not covered under the VICP. Cases involving them are heard in civil court. Preservatives and adjuvants are considered part of the vaccine, and claims against them are heard under the VICP process. The individual must produce extensive medical records to prove that the vaccine is the only thing that could have caused the alleged damage (see Chapter 4 for how VICP works).

Many anti-vaccinationists see the existence of the VICP as acknowledgment by the government that vaccines are unsafe. They suggest that the government uses the VICP as a way to limit vaccine damage claims by refusing to recognize in the VIT certain disorders such as autism that anti-vaccinationists believe are caused by vaccines and by making the documentation required to file a claim unreasonably burdensome.

Mainstream Medical Views on Vaccine Safety

The mainstream medical establishment points out that vaccines are adequately tested because every vaccine goes through three phases of clinical trials (see Chapter 4) before licensing. Dr. Paul Offit, Chief of the Division of Infectious Diseases and the Director of the Vaccine Education Center at Children's Hospital of Philadelphia, says, for example, that for rotavirus vaccine, the Phase III trial was a "placebo controlled 70,000 infant plus 11 country, 4 year, roughly $350 million study" (Wells, 2016) to assure the safety and effectiveness of the vaccine.

To do the large-scale placebo-controlled study that anti-vaccinations insist on as proof that every vaccine is safe would require tens of thousands of children to become experimental subjects. Half would be given an inoculation that contained the vaccine, the other half a placebo. Children would then be followed for years to record the diseases and disorders they contracted and their social, emotional, and physical development.

The American Medical Association and vaccine researchers believe withholding vaccine from a person at risk is a violation of medical ethics, especially when the individual does not know if he or she has been immunized as part of a study or remains vulnerable to disease from receiving a placebo. They also point to logistical problems of enrolling study subjects, asking how many parents—whether vaccine acceptors or vaccine rejectors—would allow their children to be experimented on in this way.

Many studies have examined the incidence of disorders anti-vaccinationists claim are caused by vaccines. Published peer-reviewed studies have found no significant differences between vaccinated and unvaccinated children in the development of autism, asthma, allergies, or sudden infant crib death, all of which anti-vaccinationists assert are triggered by vaccines. They also have found that the age at which a child is vaccinated makes no difference in the development of these disorders. One study that followed children to age 11 even found the vaccinated group scored significantly higher on cognitive tests than the unvaccinated group.

Many anti-vaccinationist websites have posted two studies that claim to show strong evidence that vaccinated children are less healthy than unvaccinated children. These studies have been retracted by the *Journal of Translational Science* which published them. The journal found the studies were so flawed in design, data collection, and data analysis that the results were meaningless. One significant reason for the retractions was that information on the children's vaccination status and the illnesses the child had experienced were collected by a telephone survey and relied on parental memory. No actual medical records were examined.

The medical establishment also points out that as an ongoing safety check, data about adverse events continue to be collected by a postlicensing vaccine safety surveillance system called the Vaccine Adverse Event Reporting System, to which anyone can make a report. The Vaccine Safety Data Link, the Clinical Immunization Safety Assessment Project, and the Post-Licensure Rapid Immunization Safety Monitoring also are used to detect any safety issues that may be so extremely rare as to remain unobserved in prelicensing clinical trials (see Chapter 4).

Aluminum in Vaccines

Since thimerosal has been removed from vaccines, the safety debate has turned to the adjuvant aluminum. Aluminum is *not* a heavy metal as Jenny McCarthy states. It is added to some vaccines in tiny quantities in the form of aluminum hydroxide, aluminum phosphate, or potassium aluminum sulfate (also called alum). Aluminum is also found in many over-the-counter antacids, infant formula, breast milk, some foods, and drinking water.

The amount of aluminum in vaccines is limited to 0.85–1.25 mg per dose. Following the CDC-recommended vaccination schedule for the first six months of life, a baby would be exposed to about 4 mg of aluminum, a tiny amount compared to the 10 mg a baby would be exposed to in breast milk, 40 mg in milk-based formula, or 120 mg in soy formula over the same period. Because the amount of aluminum in vaccines is very small

compared to aluminum acquired from other sources, the medical establishment sees no rationale for separate testing on aluminum exposure from
vaccines.

The Vaccine Injury Compensation Program

Almost 90 percent of adverse effects from vaccines are mild and
transient—reactions such as redness and soreness at the injection site, low
fever, and muscle aches. However, because of variability in human biology, the U.S. government recognizes that very rarely someone will have
a serious reaction to a vaccine. The most common serious adverse effects
are anaphylaxis (a life-threatening allergic response) and encephalopathy
or encephalitis (brain inflammation). The establishment of the VICP to
compensate those rare individuals that vaccines harm is considered not as
an admission that vaccines are unsafe, but as an ethical response to vulnerable individuals. Between 2006 and 2016, 3.1 billion doses of vaccines
covered under the VICP program were administered. Alleged vaccine
damage resulted in 5,407 VICP cases of which 3,661 were compensated,
the equivalent of one vaccine-injured person for every 1 million doses of
covered vaccines given.

CHAPTER 10

Do Vaccines Cause Developmental Delays?

For years anti-vaccinationist parents have claimed that vaccines damage children by causing irreversible developmental delays. They cite stories of children who received a vaccine and then days, weeks, or months later began to regress, lose skills, and show behavioral changes. According to a 2014 National Consumer League survey, about one-third of American parents believe that vaccines can cause autism spectrum disorder (ASD), often simply called autism.

Signs of autism tend to appear early in childhood at about the same time children receive multiple vaccinations. Children with ASD show a variety of symptoms and behaviors that range from mild to so severe as to be totally disabling. The disorder is characterized by

- mental and physical developmental regression; children lose skills they already have and fail to regain them;
- persistent difficulty understanding verbal and nonverbal communication to a degree that interferes with normal social and emotional relationships and social participation;
- repetitive or obsessive patterns of behavior, interests, or activities; and
- abnormal responses to environmental stimuli.

BACKGROUND: DIPHTHERIA-TETANUS-PERTUSSIS VACCINE

The diphtheria-tetanus-pertussis combination vaccine (often called DPT but referred to by the medical establishment as DTP) was licensed in the United States in 1947. The pertussis component can cause side effects, most often soreness at the injection site and short-lived high fever. However, soon after the DPT vaccine was approved, scattered but rare reports suggested that it might cause brain damage. These claims were investigated by the medical establishment and dismissed, but some people continued to question the safety of the vaccine.

In 1982, the NBC station in Washington, D.C., broadcast a program called *DPT: Vaccine Roulette* (see Chapter 6 for details on the broadcast). The program featured children who, according to their parents, showed normal, age-appropriate development before receiving DPT vaccine, but then weeks or months later experienced seizures, developmental regression, and permanent disabilities.

Barbara Loe Fisher had a son, Chris, who began to regress mentally and physically at age two-and-half. Chris had experienced a convulsion, shock, and brain inflammation after his fourth DPT shot. After seeing *DPT: Vaccine Roulette*, Fisher was convinced the shot had caused brain damage that left him with attention deficit disorder and autism.

Motivated by the belief DPT had harmed her son, Fisher contacted other parents whose children had shown similar autism-like regressions after the shot. These parents formed an organization, Dissatisfied Parents Together. Their goal was to force the government to recognize the claim that DPT vaccine had harmed their children and to eliminate vaccination as a condition for public school attendance. Formation of this organization is considered the beginning of the modern American anti-vaccination movement in the United States (see Chapter 6).

Dissatisfied Parents Together soon changed its name to the National Vaccine Information Center (NVIC) and today remains active in the anti-vaccination movement. NVIC quickly expanded to include parents who believed that many or all vaccines cause harm. Despite the name, it has no connection to any governmental organization.

The original DPT vaccine that Fisher blamed for her son's disabilities was made using whole killed bacteria. In 1997, the United States replaced the whole-cell DPT vaccine with an acellular version (DTaP). This is a subunit vaccine that uses only a few pertussis proteins, not the whole bacterium, to stimulate immunity. The change was made to reduce side effects of the vaccine, but the new vaccine has not satisfied anti-vaccination parents who continue to believe the reformulated vaccine is also unsafe.

Fisher has continued to advocate against vaccines. In 2010, she sued vaccine expert Dr. Paul Offit, author Amy Wallace, and Condé Nast publishers for libeling her in an article in *Wired* magazine. Part of the complaint was that the article "portrays those like Fisher (who oppose mandatory vaccination) as unscientific, uneducated, and harmful to society. By contrast, the article portrays Defendant Offit as a heroic pediatrician who selflessly campaigns for mandatory vaccination in a fight against enemies of science and opportunists" (U.S. District Court, 2010). The case was dismissed without being heard because the court declared there was no basis for a lawsuit. Today, NVIC claims that it is not anti-vaccine but is pro-safe vaccine. Nevertheless, Barbara Loe Fisher, the organization's president, continues to appear as a speaker at anti-vaccination events, and material on the organization's website supports anti-vaccination arguments.

Anti-Vaccinationist View of DPT/DTaP

Although the connection between autism and DTaP vaccine has been eclipsed by the endless measles vaccine–autism controversy, many anti-vaccinationists continue to believe that DTaP can cause autism, attention-deficit hyperactivity disorder, and other regressive developmental disorders. In 2016, multiple anti-vaccination websites posted articles with eye-catching headlines such as "Vaccine Maker Admits on FDA Website That DTaP Vaccine Causes Autism" (Frompovich, 2016) and "NOW IT'S OFFICIAL: FDA Announced That Vaccines Are Causing Autism!" (Vaccine Information Coalition, n.d.). The basis for these headlines was a 2005 package insert for the DTaP vaccine Tripedia that listed autism and sudden infant death syndrome (SIDS) as unverified self-reported postlicensure adverse reactions.

The connection between DPT/DTaP vaccine and SIDS is echoed by anti-vaccinationist chiropractor Brad Case. He writes "Many feel that SIDS is not some mysterious disease, but merely a deceptive label to cover up the fact that yet another child has become a victim of an adverse vaccine reaction. There are countless incidents of healthy children being vaccinated for DPT one day and their mothers finding them dead in their cribs the next morning" (Case, 2010, 256). He cites no research to support this statement, but many vaccine-skeptic parents continue to believe the vaccine is both potentially dangerous and unnecessary.

Mainstream Medical View of DPT/DTaP

The mainstream medical establishment firmly believes the benefits of DTaP far outweigh the risks, especially in children under one year old. For example, in 2016, the Centers for Disease Control and Prevention (CDC) reported 15,737 cases of pertussis in the United States. Of children younger than six months old who became infected, 44.5 percent required hospitalization. The children who were infected either had not been vaccinated or were too young to complete the series of shots needed to confer immunity.

Most reactions to DTaP are mild or moderate and transient and are much less serious than the diseases the vaccine prevents. Physicians, however, do recognize that in fewer than one in one million DTaP doses, severe reactions may occur. These reactions are anaphylaxis, encephalopathy (brain damage) or encephalitis (brain inflammation), shoulder injury related to vaccine administration, and vasovagal syncope (fainting from the body's overreactive response to a stimulus). These are the only adverse effects for DPT/DTaP listed in the Vaccine Injury Table used by the Vaccine Injury Compensation Program (see Chapter 4). Despite these rare reactions, the benefits continue to outweigh risks by preventing hundreds of hospitalizations and deaths each year.

The medical establishment does not recognize autism or SIDS as being caused by *any* vaccine. The sensational headlines that DTaP causes autism and/or SIDS come from a 13-year-old package insert for one version of DTaP. The insert lists a dozen of events including autism and SIDS that parents self-reported as occurring at some time after the vaccine was given. The insert concludes "Because these events are reported voluntarily from a population of uncertain size, it is not always possible to reliably estimate their frequencies or to establish a causal relationship to components of Tripedia vaccine" (SanofiPasteur, 2005). The same document shows that neither autism nor SIDS was found to occur during prelicensure clinical trials.

Autism researchers believe ASD is caused by the interaction of genetic mutations and exposure to environmental triggers that most likely occurs during fetal development. SIDS occurs only in infants less than one year old. Behavioral factors are thought to play a role. For example, encouraging parents to put infants to sleep on their back rather than on their stomach has decreased SIDS deaths in the United States by 58 percent since 1994. No relationship between any vaccine and SIDS has been found.

BACKGROUND: MMR VACCINE AND AUTISM

The debate over whether measles, mumps, and rubella (MMR) vaccine causes autism has lasted longer, gotten more media attention, and had a greater effect on decreasing vaccination rates than any other vaccine controversy. The debate was kicked off by gastroenterology researcher Dr. Andrew Wakefield (1957–). In England in the early 1990s, Wakefield was a member of the Inflammatory Bowel Disease (IBD) Study Group at the Royal Free Hospital in London. The group was researching the causes of ulcerative colitis and Crohn's disease. Some preliminary findings suggested that a virus along with genetic sensitivity and/or an environmental exposure might trigger Crohn's disease. Eventually, the group came to suspect that because the measles virus contained live attenuated (weakened) virus, it might possibly be a factor in the development of Crohn's disease.

While this research was under way, Wakefield began working with a few autistic children who also had serious bowel problems. He became convinced that there was a cause-and-effect connection between IBD, measles vaccine, and autism. He called this new syndrome autistic enterocolitis. In 1998, Wakefield and 12 colleagues published in *The Lancet,* a highly respected, peer-reviewed medical journal, a paper with the tongue-twisting title "Ileal-lymphoid-Nodular Hyperplasia, Non-specific Colitis, and Pervasive Developmental Disorder in Children." The researchers reported on 12 children, 8 of whom developed bowel inflammation and autism-like developmental delays that, according to the children's parents, began soon after they had received MMR vaccine. An additional child was reported to have developed similar symptoms after having naturally acquired measles.

This research would probably have gone unnoticed outside the community of gastroenterology researchers except that Wakefield publicized it by holding a news conference at which he announced that because of these research results, he could no longer support the use of MMR vaccine. In his opinion, giving three vaccines together increased the likelihood of an adverse response that could lead to autism. He identified the measles component of the vaccine as the likely culprit. Wakefield recommended children not receive MMR combination vaccine and, contrary to public health recommendations, have each component given separately at one-year intervals.

Wakefield's statements were widely publicized by British media, and fear of an MMR–autism connection drove MMR vaccination rates down in Great Britain from 92 percent in 1996 to 80 percent in 2004. In some communities, only 65 percent of children received the vaccine. The measles–autism story spread to the United States, where it was publicized by Barbara Loe Fisher and NVIC. Soon, frightened American parents were also rejecting the MMR vaccine.

ANTI-VACCINATIONIST VIEW OF AN MMR VACCINE–AUTISM CONNECTION

To members of the anti-vaccination community with autistic children, Andrew Wakefield is a misunderstood hero whose work has been suppressed by the medical establishment and pharmaceutical companies because it challenges mainstream views. For these families, Wakefield's argument that MMR vaccine can trigger autism offers an explanation for the disorder and a possible path to treatment. Because Wakefield was a medical doctor and *The Lancet* a reputable journal, some members of the anti-vaccination community continue to believe his assertions and believe that he is unjustly maligned.

Six years after the controversial Wakefield paper was published, Brian Deer, a British investigative journalist, went to *The Lancet* with information that the research detailed in the 1998 Wakefield paper had been conducted unethically. He claimed that the children in the study were preselected and referred to Wakefield by attorneys who planned to represent their families in lawsuits against the vaccine manufacturer. He also claimed that Wakefield was paid more than Ł400,000 (about $912,000 in 2018 dollars) by the attorneys to perform the study that led to his MMR–autism conclusion. Wakefield had not disclosed this conflict of interest to the hospital, his colleagues, or *The Lancet*.

Deer's investigation eventually caused *The Lancet* to declare Wakefield's research fraudulent and to retract the paper. However, almost 15 years later, Wakefield and his supporters continue to dismiss Deer's findings. They claim Deer was paid by a pharmaceutical industry group interested in discrediting Wakefield's research and that Deer sensationalized the story and maligned Wakefield to further his own journalistic career. In 2017, anti-vaccinationist and pharmaceutical industry skeptic Vera Sharav published a long article on the Alliance for Human Research Protection website claiming Deer's findings, which resulted in Wakefield losing his medical license in the United Kingdom in 2010, were completely bogus and without merit and that Wakefield's research was unfairly targeted.

Wakefield continues to defend himself. In his autobiography, *Callous Disregard: Autism and Vaccines—The Truth behind a Tragedy,* he claims the charges against him were politically motivated. In 2012, he filed a defamation lawsuit in Texas against Brian Deer, *BMJ*, a British medical journal that published a second set of charges by Deer, and Fiona Godlee, its editor. The suit was dismissed, and Wakefield was ordered to pay the defendant's costs. He has also continued to claim that in multiple cases, "the government themselves have conceded that the vaccine [MMR] cause the autism" (Age of Autism, 2013).

Wakefield and anti-vaccinationist Barbara Loe Fisher still find an audience for their beliefs that vaccines cause developmental delays. They were keynote speakers at the 2014 International Chiropractic Pediatric Association convention. Wakefield also cowrote and directed the 2016 film *Vaxxed: From Cover-up to Catastrophe*. In it, he and anti-vaccinationist

Brian Hooper claim scientists at the CDC covered up and destroyed evidence from a study that showed a connection between autism and MMR vaccine (see Chapter 13 for more on conspiracy theories). When *Newsweek* asked Wakefield if he still believed the MMR vaccine causes autism, his answer was "Yes, I do. I think MMR contributes to the current autism epidemic" (Ziv, 2015). Many anti-vaccinationists agree with him.

Mainstream Medical View of an MMR Vaccine–Autism Connection

In the mainstream medical establishment's view, there is absolutely no connection between MMR vaccine, measles virus, and autism. To the medical establishment, there is no controversy or reason to question the vaccine. MMR does not trigger autism. It considers Wakefield at best pigheaded and misguided and at worst a fraud who plays on parents' fears.

In the interpretation section of the paper that started this controversy, the authors said that they had "identified associated gastrointestinal disease and developmental regression in a group of previously normal children, which was generally associated in time with possible environmental triggers" (Wakefield et al., 1998). They *did not* say that measles or measles vaccine caused developmental delays, only that a connection appeared possible. When Wakefield defended his public statement that measles vaccine causes developmental delays, 10 of the 12 coauthors of the paper produced a written statement saying Wakefield had gone too far in making assumptions and drawing conclusions that were not supported by the research data.

Dozens of studies by scientists at other institutions worldwide have failed to find an MMR–autism link. For example, one study looked at 500 children diagnosed with autism who had received MMR vaccine at different times during childhood. Researchers found no increased onset of autism soon after vaccination regardless of the age at which the vaccine was administered. They also looked back in medical records for a spike in autism diagnoses after the MMR vaccine was introduced and found no rapid increase. Research from Japan where the MMR combination vaccine was discontinued in 1993 in favor of individual shots has shown no decrease in autism diagnoses after the switch to individual shots. Multiple other international studies failed to find any connection between MMR vaccine and autism.

After investigative journalist Brian Deer produced evidence that convinced *The Lancet* that Wakefield's research was fatally flawed and caused the journal to retract the paper, the British General Medical Council began hearings on Wakefield's fitness to practice medicine due to charges of professional misconduct. On May 24, 2010, Wakefield lost his license to practice medicine in the United Kingdom.

Brian Deer, who says he was paid by London's *Sunday Times* and not by any pharmaceutical organization, continued to investigate Wakefield's research. He discovered Wakefield had filed a patent application in June 1997 before the controversial research paper was published. The patent was for a new vaccine/immunization to prevent measles with a therapeutic component to treat IBD and autism. It appeared from the filing that Wakefield intended to profit from what he called autistic enterocolitis by offering a new measles vaccine.

In 2011, Deer published an article claiming that medical information about the children in the 1998 study had been altered, that three of the nine children who were reported to have regressive autism did not have an autism diagnosis at all, and that although all the children were declared to have been developmentally normal before receiving the MMR vaccine, five of them had documented developmental problems before inoculation.

Dr. Paul Offit, director of the Vaccine Education Center at Children's Hospital of Philadelphia, sums up the controversy this way: "This was a collection of . . . 8 children who had autism within months of receiving MMR . . . I mean, you frankly could have published a paper claiming that peanut butter sandwiches caused leukemia because you had 8 children who recently for the first time in their life ate peanut butter sandwiches and then developed leukemia. You have to have a higher bar than that" (Wells, 2018). There is no MMR–measles virus–autism connection.

BACKGROUND: MERCURY IN VACCINES AND AUTISM

Thimerosal is a compound used in small quantities since the 1930s to keep some vaccines, ophthalmic solutions, nasal solutions, and tattoo inks free of bacterial and fungal contamination. In the 1990s, it became the most controversial component of vaccines because it is 49.5 percent organic mercury by weight. Mercury is a recognized neurotoxin (nerve poison). The expression "mad as a hatter" comes from behavioral changes such as irritability, depression, extreme shyness, and insomnia that were observed centuries ago in hat makers in England who were exposed to mercury compounds during the preparation of felt. Prolonged mercury exposure also causes tremors, delusions, hallucinations, and memory loss.

Humans are exposed to mercury in two main forms, methylmercury and ethylmercury. Today, most human exposure comes from burning coal to generate electricity, volcanic eruptions, and forest fires. Rain and dust bring mercury down out of the atmosphere and deposit it in oceans and waterways. Bacteria in the water convert it into methylmercury. Other organisms eat the bacteria, and methylmercury enters the food chain. Methylmercury is poorly eliminated and builds up in tissue, so that at each step in the food chain, its concentration increases. Pregnant and breast-feeding women are advised to avoid eating swordfish, tuna, and other fish near the top of the food chain because they may contain enough methyl-mercury to harm the unborn child or breastfeeding infant.

In the body, thimerosal breaks down into two compounds, thiosalicylate and ethylmercury. Ethylmercury is different from methylmercury. Unlike methylmercury, ethylmercury is chemically broken down and eliminated from the body in feces. It is highly unlikely to accumulate to harmful levels.

Questions about thimerosal in vaccines arose in 1997 when Congress passed the Food and Drug Modernization Act, an update of the 1938 Federal Food, Drug, and Cosmetic Act. One directive in the new Act required the Food and Drug Administration (FDA) to evaluate the effect of mercury on humans. This requirement was added as an amendment by a senator from New Jersey. He had no interest in vaccines but was concerned about methylmercury accumulation in fish. Following the law's directive, the FDA compiled a list of foods and drugs to be evaluated. Vaccines containing thimerosal were on that list.

In 1999, the FDA concluded that a six-month-old child could receive a maximum of 187.5 μm of mercury from thimerosal-containing vaccines following the vaccination schedule recommended at that time. This exceeded the Environmental Protection Agency's (EPA) acceptable exposure level. The EPA did not distinguish between exposure to methylmercury and exposure to ethylmercury.

Because of the EPA's findings, the FDA sent a letter to vaccine manufacturers requesting that as a preventative measure they stop using thimerosal in vaccines. The American Academy of Pediatrics, the CDC, and the U.S. Public Health Service all supported this request. Nevertheless, for unclear reasons, instead of pushing forward in requiring thimerosal-free vaccines, the FDA backed off and began issuing statements claiming that there was no convincing evidence that thimerosal caused harm. This was problematic, as at the time few studies had compared the metabolism of methylmercury and ethylmercury. Those that did exist had been done on animals. The FDA was forced to admit that no one had looked at how ethylmercury might affect babies in the womb or infants. Then in 2000, Congress got involved and mercury in vaccines became a topic of widespread public debate.

Congressman Dan Burton, a conservative Republican from Indiana, called hearings on the relationship between vaccines, mercury, and autism. He had a personal interest in the vaccine–autism question. His grandson was autistic. He freely acknowledged his grandson's disorder, but he did not reveal to his colleagues or the public that he had a personal conflict of interest. His daughter had filed a petition for monetary damages in Vaccine Court. Autism was not recognized by the Vaccine Injury Table as a vaccine-caused disorder, but it appeared that Burton, using the alleged mercury–autism connection, hoped to have it added.

The Burton hearings went on for three years during which time dozens of ordinary people came before the committee to tell stories of how their normal children had developed autism soon after vaccination. Burton blasted physicians for not explaining the dangers of vaccines to their patients. The FDA and the Institute of Medicine (IOM) came under fire for not moving aggressively to remove thimerosal from vaccines. In some cases, Burton implied these agencies were covering up what he absolutely believed was the truth—that mercury in vaccines caused autism.

The hearings ended without autism being declared a vaccine-caused disorder, but the debate was far from over. Robert Kennedy, Jr., a politically connected activist, took up the cause, and as of 2018 continues to be a leader in insisting that mercury in vaccines causes autism and other disorders. Meanwhile, vaccine manufacturers began to eliminate mercury as a preservative in vaccines. Most vaccines were thimerosal-free by 2003. Today, all vaccines routinely recommended for children under six years old in the United States contain either no thimerosal or only a trace (less than 1 μm per dose) that remains from the manufacturing process; no thimerosal is added as a preservative. Some influenza vaccines and vaccines packaged in multidose vials for international use continue to contain thimerosal, but a thimerosal-free version of influenza vaccine became available in the United States in 2015.

Anti-Vaccinationist View of Mercury in Vaccines

When the mercury–vaccine–autism debate was at its peak in 2005, St. Martin's Press, a mainstream New York publisher, released *Evidence of Harm: Mercury in Vaccines and the Autism Epidemic: A Medical Controversy* by journalist David Kirby. The book related the struggles of a group that called themselves the Mercury Moms who were convinced that the mercury from thimerosal in vaccines had caused their children's autism. Discounting the fact that it is impossible with one hundred percent certainty to prove a negative, the author made the argument that because scientists could not absolutely prove there was no connection between vaccines, mercury, and autism, a connection was highly possible and even probable. The book received major publicity, and the argument for a mercury–vaccine–autism connection was promoted by autism organizations such as Autism Speaks, AutismOne, and SafeMinds.

Robert F. Kennedy, Jr., soon became one of the most vocal supporters of the mercury–vaccine–autism theory. In 2005, *Rolling Stone* magazine published an article by Kennedy titled "Deadly Immunity." The article claimed that the government deliberately covered up information showing mercury in vaccines was poisoning children and leading to an epidemic of autism. The story relied heavily on work by autism activist Dr. Mark Geier. Geier frequently testified as an expert witness in Vaccine Court that vaccines caused autism.

During the next decade, the mercury–vaccines–autism connection was the subject of intense research, costing millions of dollars and involving the medical records of thousands of children. Overwhelmingly, the research found no connection. Some autism organizations such as Autism Speaks began to walk back their position that there was a cause-and-effect connection, while others such as SafeMinds and Generation Rescue continued to insist mercury in vaccines was an autism trigger.

After mercury had been removed from childhood vaccines for more than a decade, Kennedy continued to support the mercury–vaccine–autism theory in his 2014 book *Thimerosal: Let Science Speak.* His position today is that mercury in vaccines causes a multitude of disorders including, "attention disorders, speech delays, language delays, Tourette Syndrome, misery disorder, seizures, epilepsy, sudden infant death syndrome, narcolepsy, heart disorders, neurological disorders, asthma and allergies" (Kennedy, 2016).

Kennedy is not alone in his beliefs. The 2015 documentary film *Trace Amounts* tells the story of Eric Gladen, an adult who is convinced that he was poisoned by mercury in a tetanus shot in 2004 at age 29. The film includes interviews with prominent vaccination skeptics such as retired congressman Dan Burton, researcher Brian Hooker, journalist David Kirby, and father and son Mark and David Geier. Robert Kennedy, Jr., endorsed the film and appeared at some events where it was shown.

That in 2018 all routine childhood vaccines in the United States now contain either no thimerosal or less than 1 μm per dose as a production residue does not appease vaccine skeptics who continue to insist that there is a mercury–vaccine–autism connection. These individuals claim that *any* exposure to mercury in *any* form, no matter how small, presents an unacceptable health risk to children, and therefore, to keep children safe, most vaccines should be avoided.

Despite all the evidence against an MMR–autism connection, the idea remains so entrenched in the minds of some members of the British public that in 2018 the British Veterinary Association issued a statement that canine vaccines did not cause autism in dogs. In fact, dogs do not ever develop autism.

MAINSTREAM MEDICAL VIEW OF MERCURY IN VACCINES

The mainstream medical view is that ethylmercury in the form of thimerosal in vaccines is not and never was a trigger for autism. The CDC states, "The evidence is clear: thimerosal is not a toxin in vaccines" (CDC, 2013) and goes on to cite multiple large, well-documented studies to support this conclusion. The IOM looked specifically at whether thimerosal-containing vaccines were related to autism and concluded, "the body of epidemiological evidence favors rejection of a causal relationship between thimerosal-containing vaccines and autism" (IOM, 2004). WHO's Global Vaccine Advisory Committee on Vaccine Safety agrees with this position. Even Autism Speaks now accepts the IOM conclusion that there is no connection and states in its policy on autism and mercury: "The body of evidence gathered through epidemiologic research to date does not currently support a causal relationship between thimerosal in childhood vaccines and autism risk" (Autism Speaks, 2018). In addition, many of the arguments for a vaccine–autism connection presented in David Kirby's book *Evidence of Harm* were refuted by Seth Mnookin who explored the alleged connection in his book *The Panic Virus* published by Simon & Schuster in 2011.

Even though only miniscule traces of thimerosal have been present in a few select vaccines for the past 15 years, the rate of autism has continued to rise. Thimerosal was removed from vaccines in Europe in 1992, almost a decade before it was taken out of vaccines in the United States, yet when researchers in Denmark and Sweden compared the rate of autism in children vaccinated before thimerosal was removed and those immunized with thimerosal-free vaccines, they found "a relatively stable incidence of autism when thimerosal-containing vaccines were in use (1980–1990), including years when children were exposed to as much as 200 µg of ethylmercury . . . However, in 1990, a steady increase in the incidence of autism began in both countries and continued [from 1990–2000] despite the removal of thimerosal from vaccines in 1992" (Plotkin, 2009). This strongly suggests something other than vaccines has caused the rapid increase in autism diagnoses.

Additional evidence that there is no thimerosal–autism connection comes from the fact that children with mercury poisoning show muscle, speech, sensory, psychiatric, visual, and other signs that are either different from or absent in children with autism. Alternately, children with rare disorders such as Dravet syndrome, West syndrome, Ohtahara syndrome, Lennox-Gastaut syndrome, and Landau-Kleffner syndrome develop seizures, chronic illness, and autism-like developmental delays. These signs, which could be mistaken for autism, appear in early childhood at the same time in both vaccinated and unvaccinated children. Little is known about the cause of some of these disorders, but Dravet syndrome is attributed to a mutation in the *SCN1A* gene, not to vaccine administration.

What about the activists who continue to support the theory that thimerosal triggers autism? Many of the claims they cite have been shown to be fraudulent or come from studies conducted without scientific rigor and appropriate peer review. For example, *Rolling Stone* was forced to completely retract Kennedy's "Deadly Immunity" story. The piece had relied heavily on suspect work by autism activist Dr. Mark Geier. Geier lost his license to practice medicine in 2011 for using unapproved medical and alternative treatments to "cure" autism at the clinic he and his son ran in Maryland. However, he continues to perform private research on the mercury–vaccine–autism connection, and his papers continue to be cited by anti-vaccinationists such as the makers of the *Trace Amounts* film.

To the mainstream medical world, the large number of high-quality studies that have tested the mercury–vaccine–autism theory have shown conclusively that there is no relationship between thimerosal in vaccines and autism or any other disorder. Vaccine expert Dr. Stanley Plotkin sums up the mainstream viewpoint this way: "These studies [of MMR vaccine and thimerosal] have been performed in several countries by many different investigators who have employed a multitude of epidemiologic and statistical methods. The large size of the studied populations has afforded a level of statistical power sufficient to detect even rare associations" (Plotkin, 2009).

CHAPTER 11

Is the Government-Recommended Vaccination Schedule Appropriate?

Only 2 to 4 percent of American parents reject all vaccines, but about 30 percent are vaccine skeptics. Vaccine-skeptic parents question the validity of the vaccination schedule recommended by the U.S. Centers for Disease Control and Prevention (CDC). They choose to deviate from the schedule by refusing vaccines that they decide are too risky or are unnecessary, and/or they change the timing of vaccine administration. This has led to popularization of so called alternative vaccine schedules to address these parents' concerns. The mainstream medical establishment contends that alternative schedules provide no benefits, unnecessarily leave children vulnerable to vaccine-preventable diseases, and that the best way to keep children healthy is to follow the CDC schedule.

BACKGROUND: VACCINATING SELECTIVELY

Every year, the CDC releases a recommended immunization schedule based on a review of vaccine data by the Advisory Committee on Immunization Practices (ACIP). ACIP members are vaccine experts. To prevent bias, they cannot be employed by a vaccine manufacturer or hold a patent on a vaccine. They are permitted to be involved in vaccine studies but cannot vote on the vaccine they are studying, on any other vaccine manufactured by a company funding their research, or on any similar vaccine manufactured by a different company.

The ACIP schedule considers the age at which each vaccine should be administered, number of doses needed to achieve immunity, optimal time between doses, frequency and severity of the disease, frequency and severity of adverse effects, precautions to be observed, and recommendations on who should not be vaccinated. The schedule is the medically preferred schedule for healthy American children from birth to age 18. It begins with newborn vaccination against hepatitis B. By age six, children will have received 32–34 inoculations giving them immunity against 10 diseases, some of which will require booster shots later in childhood. By age 18, following the standard schedule, an individual will have been vaccinated against three additional diseases.

ACIP's recommendations are only recommendations. The American Medical Association, American Academy of Pediatrics (AAP), the American Academy of Family Physicians, the American College of Obstetricians and Gynecologists, and the American College of Nurse-Midwives strongly support following the CDC schedule, but there is no legal requirement to do so. Individual physicians and parents may choose to alter or ignore the schedule. Table 11.1 outlines childhood inoculations by the age at which they are recommended for healthy children.

The adult CDC-recommended vaccine schedule emphasizes booster shots such as Td, Tdap, and influenza to maintain immunity initiated in childhood. It also adds vaccines against shingles and pneumococcal disease for older adults. Several vaccines such as hepatitis A and hepatitis B did not exist when many older adults were children, so some adults have not received these vaccines. These adults may be vaccinated if they or their physician feel vaccination would be beneficial. Likewise, individuals who were not fully vaccinated as children or who did not have the natural diseases prevented by MMR and varicella vaccine can be vaccinated as adults. The percentage of fully vaccinated adults is much lower than that of children. Table 11.2 summarizes common adult vaccines and percentage of coverage.

Table 11.1 Recommended Schedule of Vaccine Doses for Healthy Children Birth to Age 18 Years

Vaccine	Timing of Administration	Doses before Age 18
Hepatitis B	birth, 1 month, 6 months	3
Rotavirus	2 and 4 months (2-dose series)	2 or 3
	2, 4, and 6 months (3-dose series)	
Diphtheria, Tetanus, Pertussis (DTaP)	4, 6, and 15–18 months and 4–6 years with additional booster shots of T and D every 10 years	5
Haemophilus influenzae type b (Hib)	2, 4, and 12–15 months (3-dose series) 2, 4, 6, and 12–15 months (4-dose series)	3 or 4

Vaccine	Timing of Administration	Doses before Age 18
Inactivated polio (IPV)	2, 4, 6–18 months, and 4–6 years	4
Pneumococcal PCV13	2, 4, 6, and 12–15 months	4
Influenza	6 months with a second dose at 7 months followed by single dose every year in the autumn	18
Mumps, measles, and rubella	12–15 months and 4–6 years	2
Varicella	12–15 months and 4–6 years	2
Hepatitis A	12–23 months with second dose six months later	2
Human Papillomavirus (HPV)	11–12 years with second dose 2 months later for children who receive the first dose between ages 11–14; a third dose is needed 6 months from the first dose for individuals who receive their first dose between ages 15–26	2 or 3
Meningococcal strains A, C, W, Y	11–12 years and 16 years	2
Meningococcal strain B	16 years followed by a second dose 1 month later (2-dose series) 16 years followed by doses at 1 month and 6 months (3-dose series)	2 or 3

Note: Vaccines are listed by the approximate age at which they are recommended.

Based on the 2018 CDC-recommended schedule for healthy children. Recommendations will vary for at-risk subpopulations. Parents of children with impaired health should consult their pediatrician before vaccinating.

Source: https://www.cdc.gov/vaccines/schedules/hcp/child-adolescent.html.

Table 11.2 Recommended Schedule of Vaccine Doses for Adults

Vaccine	Timing of Administration	Total Doses	Percentage of Adults Vaccinated in 2016
Influenza	Once every year in early autumn	Varies with lifespan	43.5% 2016–17 season
Td	Every 10 years throughout life except when Tdap is given	Varies with lifespan	62.2% in last 10 years
Tdap	Women weeks 27–36 of each pregnancy; others once per adult lifetime	One time for everyone and once during each pregnancy for women	26.6% total adult population
Hepatitis A	Any time with second dose 6 weeks later	2	9.5%

(Continued)

Table 11.2 (Continued)

Vaccine	Timing of Administration	Total Doses	Percentage of Adults Vaccinated in 2016
Hepatitis B	Any time with second dose 1 month after the first and third dose 6 months after the first	3	24.8%
Herpes zoster (shingles)	60 years or older	1 or 2	33.4%
PCV13/PPSV23	65 years with PPSV23 booster every 5 years	Varies with lifespan	24.0%

Note: Vaccines are listed by the approximate age at which they are recommended.

Based on the 2018 CDC-recommended schedule for healthy adults who have received all recommended childhood vaccinations available at the time of their childhood.

Recommendations will vary for at-risk subpopulations. Individuals with health concerns should consult their physician before vaccinating.

Sources: https://www.cdc.gov/vaccines/imz-managers/coverage/adultvaxview/NHIS-2016.html and https://www.cdc.gov/vaccines/schedules/hcp/imz/adult.html

ANTI-VACCINATIONIST VIEW ON SELECTIVE VACCINATION

"Why are we giving our children so many vaccines?" asks Jennifer Margolis, a well-educated vaccine skeptic interviewed in the 2010 *Frontline* documentary "The Vaccine War." "There's no more polio in the United States, and there's no more diphtheria. When do we take polio off the vaccine schedule?" (Public Broadcasting System, 2010).

The last case of native polio occurred in the United States in 1979. Native measles also has been eliminated, although infected travelers periodically import the disease. Cases of diphtheria are rare. Because these diseases are unusual in the developed world, vaccine skeptics think that to immunize against them is to take an unnecessary risk. They believe their children will be protected by herd immunity because other parents have vaccinated their children.

The perception also exists among vaccine skeptics that certain childhood diseases such as chickenpox and rotavirus are not serious enough to vaccinate against. Margolis, whose children did not receive the chickenpox vaccine, sums up that outlook on the disease this way: "As a parent, I would rather see my child get a natural illness and contract it the way illnesses have been contracted for at least 200,000 years. I'm not afraid of my child getting chickenpox. . . Getting sick is not a bad thing" (Public Broadcasting System, 2010).

The most widely publicized schedule for eliminating certain vaccines is Dr. Bob's Selective Vaccination Schedule. Dr. Bob is Southern California pediatrician Robert Sears. He lays out his selective vaccination schedule in *The Vaccine Book: Making the Right Decision for Your Child* published in 2007 and updated in 2011.

Dr. Bob's selective schedule is designed for parents who want to avoid vaccines they consider risky or unnecessary. The schedule starts at two months with DTaP and rotavirus, but it eliminates all inoculations against polio, mumps, measles, rubella, and hepatitis A. It delays the hepatitis B vaccine (normally recommended for newborns) until age 12–14 years and recommends antigen (blood) testing for 10-year-olds to determine if the child has acquired natural immunity to mumps, measles, rubella, chicken-pox, and hepatitis A. If the child has not had these, Sears suggests parents consider vaccinating against them before puberty because these diseases cause more serious symptoms in teens and adults than in young children.

The Sears Selective Vaccination Schedule is not the most extreme alternative schedule. Donald Miller, a physician and professor of surgery, recommends no vaccinations at all until age two years. His theory is that by age two, the brain is 80 percent developed and is less likely to be harmed by vaccines. He believes the risk of DTaP outweighs any benefits and that no live attenuated vaccines (i.e., MMR, chickenpox, and rotavirus) should ever be given. He recommends all inoculations be spaced at six-month intervals. A few other physicians have also developed selective schedules based on their own beliefs about vaccine safety and utility.

MAINSTREAM MEDICAL VIEW ON SELECTIVE VACCINATION

The mainstream medical community maintains that compliance with the CDC vaccination schedule protects individuals from becoming ill and communities from experiencing outbreaks of potentially life-threatening vaccine-preventable diseases. Although developed countries have significantly reduced the incidence of vaccine-preventable illness, travelers coming from other countries can import these diseases during an incubation period during which they are contagious but do not show significant signs of illness.

Diseases vaccine-skeptic parents think their children will never encounter flourish in war zones, in refugee camps, during natural disasters, and in countries with few immunization laws and poor immunization outreach. Wild polio still exists in 2018 in Afghanistan and Pakistan; however, other countries, mostly in Africa and Southeast Asia but also Ukraine, Syria, Yemen, and Iraq, are considered at continued risk for polio outbreaks. Only one or two cases of diphtheria occur in the United States and Canada each year, but 35 countries reported diphtheria outbreaks in 2016. India topped the list with more than 3,380 cases and Madagascar had 2,865. Developed countries such as Australia, Austria, France, Germany, Spain, and the United Kingdom all reported diphtheria cases. European countries reported more than 14,000 measles cases with 34 deaths in the first six months of 2017, and between 2010 and 2015, there were between 18,700 and 48,300 cases of pertussis every year in the United States.

Although vaccine-skeptic parents view chickenpox and rotavirus as relatively benign childhood diseases, rotavirus, which causes severe diarrhea and dehydration, is responsible for 215,000 deaths worldwide each year. Chickenpox usually is mild in a healthy child, but if a child spreads chickenpox to a person whose immune system is compromised by cancer treatment, an organ transplant, or an immune-suppressing disease such as HIV/AIDS, the result can be deadly.

People with weakened immune systems cannot be safely vaccinated against chickenpox or measles because they contain live attenuated virus. These people tend to have a much more severe responses to infection than healthy individuals. These diseases can also have serious health consequences if contracted by adults. Mainstream medical and public health organizations support full, on-time vaccination as the best way to protect both individuals and the community from diseases that are far more likely to cause serious health complications than vaccine administration.

BACKGROUND: VACCINE SCHEDULING

In the past 30 years, new vaccines for children under age six years have been added to the recommended schedule. This has led to the practice of administering more than one vaccine at a single well child visit and the development of combination vaccines to reduce the number of shots a child receives. It has also created a movement by vaccine-skeptic parents to spread out or delay vaccinations.

The idea that combination vaccines are more harmful than individual vaccines started when Andrew Wakefield (see Chapter 10) claimed (falsely) in a press conference that he could no longer support the use of the combination MMR vaccine because he believed receiving three vaccines at once increased the chance of a child developing autism. He advocated for each vaccine to be given separately at one-year intervals.

Since then, the number of combination vaccines has grown. As many as five vaccines can be combined in a single shot, for example DTaP-IPV-Hib (Pentacel) or DTaP-IP-Hep B (Pediarix). Even if combination vaccines are not used, it is common to give more than one individual vaccine at a single office visit. The most common type of vaccine resistance that mainstream pediatricians encounter is parents asking to alter the recommended vaccination schedule by spacing out and delaying certain shots.

Alternative and selective vaccination schedules frustrate mainstream pediatricians and the AAP, which see no benefit in them for healthy children. Some pediatricians feel pressured into agreeing to alternative schedules in the belief that partial or delayed vaccination is better than no vaccination. Other pediatric practices refuse to take new patients who want to alter the CDC schedule or skip some vaccinations completely. Vaccine-skeptic parents believe they are being prudent by reducing what they see as vaccination risks, while physicians feel their years of education and clinical practice are being ignored in favor of suspect internet information and what anti-vaccination activist Jenny McCarthy calls the University of Google.

Anti-Vaccinationist View on Vaccine Scheduling

Many parents feel they should have a voice in determining what medical treatments are best for their child. Vaccine-skeptic parents believe vaccination is less risky if they can spread out their child's inoculations so that the child receives only one vaccine at a time with a month or more interval between shots. This belief arises from the idea that a young child's immune system cannot handle the challenge of being exposed to so many antigens at one time. They also express concern that combination vaccines or giving more than one vaccine per office visit increases health risks by increasing a child's exposure to other vaccine components. Aluminum is most often the component of concern (see Chapter 9).

Some vaccine-skeptic parents believe that combination vaccines do not work as well as individual shots or that the individual vaccines in a combination shot interact in a way that harms their child. J. B. Handley, father of a child with autism and founder of Generation Rescue, an anti-vaccine autism organization, told *Frontline* that at a single office visit, "my kid got six vaccines. You don't have any science that can show me that the regression [to autism] wasn't triggered by the six vaccines" (Public Broadcasting System, 2010). Parents who object to the CDC schedule believe that they are vaccinating in a way that poses the least risk to their child.

Another vaccine-skeptic scheduling issue arises specifically over vaccines against hepatitis B and human papillomavirus (HPV). Hepatitis B is a highly contagious liver disease transmitted by contact with body fluids containing the virus. Most cases of hepatitis B are sexually transmitted, although the disease can also be passed by accidental contact with infected blood or when a baby passes through the birth canal of an infected mother. The CDC recommendation is to vaccinate newborns against hepatitis B before they leave the hospital. Vaccine-skeptic parents find this ridiculous, as their baby will not be sexually active for years. They believe immunization of a newborn unnecessarily stresses its immune system.

HPV is a group of very common sexually transmitted viruses that can cause genital warts and genital cancers in both men and women. The CDC recommends vaccinating children at age 11 years, but the vaccine can be given as early as age 9. Parents, especially those who believe in sexual abstinence before marriage, protest that their child will not be sexually active for years and that receiving this vaccine at the start of puberty may encourage early sexual activity.

An increasing number of parents who are willing to vaccinate but hesitant about the CDC schedule are insisting that their pediatrician follow an alternative schedule. Dr. Bob's Alternative Vaccination Schedule is one popular schedule designed for parents who are concerned about their child receiving too many vaccines at once too early in life. Dr. Bob's schedule spaces out and delays most vaccinations when compared to the CDC schedule. It avoids hepatitis B vaccination at birth, moving it to 2.5 years and begins with DTaP and rotavirus at 2 months. After that, it recommends no more than two inoculations per visit in months 3 through 7 and at 9, 12, 15, 18, and 21 months. More vaccines are given at 2, 2.5, 3, 4, 5, 6, 7, 8, 9, 12, 13, and 16 years. In addition, annual influenza shots are recommended each year, starting at 9 months. The primary goal of this schedule is to avoid what Sears calls chemical overload.

MAINSTREAM MEDICAL VIEW ON VACCINE SCHEDULING

Mainstream pediatricians and medical organizations see no benefit and much potential harm in skipping or delaying any inoculations. They point out that no research has been done on the safety or effectiveness of alternative schedules. They are, as even Dr. Bob admits, based on the beliefs and experience of individual doctors, not on studies by vaccine experts.

It should be noted that charges were brought against Dr. Sears in September 2016 by the Medical Board of California that could result in the loss of his license to practice medicine. The charges included keeping inadequate and inaccurate medical records, gross negligence for failing to order neurological tests for a two-year-old who had been hit on the head with a hammer, and improperly exempting the same child from all future vaccinations. Since then, a second parent has filed additional complaints with the Medical Board.

Supporters of Sears claim that these charges targeted Dr. Bob because the Medical Board of California wanted to make an example of him for campaigning against a 2015 California bill that eliminated all personal and religious exemptions from vaccination. (The bill passed.) On June 27, 2018, the Medical Board put Dr. Sears on probation for the charges of alleged medical negligence and writing inappropriate medical vaccination exemptions. The Board required Sears to receive additional medical education and to be supervised by an independent physician for 35 months. Failure to meet these requirements would result in revocation of his license to practice medicine.

Mainstream pediatricians reject alternative schedules and consider the CDC schedule the fastest way to complete immunization coverage, although they will adjust the CDC schedule on an individual basis for children who are either temporarily or chronically ill. However, parents who space out or delay certain vaccines, for example, Hib, out of the belief that they are protecting their child leave the child vulnerable to disease for a longer period. In many cases, the time of increased vulnerability coincides with the time when a child is most susceptible to be seriously harmed by the disease.

A child's immune system is not fully mature at birth, but it still functions incredibly well. As soon as a baby emerges from the womb, its immune system must fight off thousands of new antigens from bacteria, fungi, viruses, and allergens that are in the air the child breathes and in virtually everything the child touches or eats. Thanks to the development subunit vaccines that use only a few proteins from the coat of a pathogen to stimulate immunity (see Chapter 2), the antigen load in vaccines, even combination vaccines, is much smaller than the environmental antigen load the child successfully manages daily. By age two, a child following the CDC schedule is exposed to only about 150 additional antigens from vaccines.

Combination vaccines reduce the number of shots a child receives. To win regulatory approval, combination vaccines must be tested to show that one component does not increase or decrease the effectiveness of another component. When several inoculations are given at the same time, these also are studied to assure that no unintended interactions occur. Compared to selective vaccination schedules, giving more than one vaccine at an office visit or using a combination vaccine substantially reduces the number of office visits needed to achieve complete coverage. The more office visits needed, the higher the cost, the higher the parental time investment, and the more likely parents will skip inoculations and fail to complete a vaccine series.

As for the timing of hepatitis B vaccination, the mainstream medical establishment believes that vaccination at birth causes no harm to the baby and presents an opportunity to improve public health and potentially eliminate hepatitis B in developed countries. Before the recommendation for newborn vaccination, about 10,000 children each year contracted hepatitis B through nonsexual contact before age 10. There is also concern that some parents who wait to vaccinate against hepatitis B will never get around having their child vaccinated, not because they object to the vaccine, but because arranging to have child vaccinated against this relatively unfamiliar disease becomes a low priority.

HPV viruses are the most common sexually transmitted viruses in the world. They infect both men and women, and there is no test to determine one's infection status. The HPV vaccine is only effective before an individual becomes sexually active; once infected, it is too late to vaccinate. The reasoning behind vaccinating at age 11 is that the vaccine will protect the child in the future whenever he or she becomes sexually active.

Dr. Kristin Feemster, research director at the Vaccine Education Center at Children's Hospital of Philadelphia, sums up the mainstream attitude toward altering the CDC vaccination schedule: "The choice to forego or delay vaccination is not just a choice between a vaccine and no vaccine; it is between a vaccine and being susceptible to a vaccine-preventable disease" (Ashland Child, 2018).

CHAPTER 12

Should Vaccination Be Mandatory?

Different countries approach the question of compulsory vaccination in different ways. In Australia, vaccination is voluntary, but the government encourages it by withholding certain government benefits from families who refuse to vaccinate and gives tax breaks to low-income families who keep their children's vaccinations current. Slovenia fines the unvaccinated. In Pakistan, failing to vaccinate children can lead to a jail sentence.

Until recently, Europe leaned toward voluntary immunization or lax enforcement of compulsory vaccination laws. However, between January 2017 and June 2017, 18 European countries reported a total of more than 14,000 measles cases with 34 deaths. This stimulated new mandatory laws and incentives in several countries. Italy accounted for 37 percent of cases in the first six months of 2017 and consequently made vaccination mandatory for daycare, preschool, and public school attendance with no personal belief or religious exemptions. In France, where only the DTaP vaccine was mandatory and 8 other vaccines recommended, children born after January 1, 2018, must now receive 11 compulsory vaccines. German parents who cannot prove they have received vaccine counseling from a doctor can be fined up to €2,500 ($2,800), and schools are required to report noncomplying parents to government health authorities.

The United States has a long history of requiring vaccinations for school entry. Those requirements have gradually extended to include daycare and preschool programs. Certain workplaces may also require adults to receive specific vaccines in the interest of public health.

BACKGROUND

In 1809, Boston became the first American city to pass a mandatory vaccination law. The law was an attempt to stop an outbreak of smallpox. Other cities in the state soon followed. In 1852, Massachusetts also became the first state to provide free public education to all children and to make school attendance compulsory. Schools became a prime setting for the spread of contagious diseases.

Public health officials quickly recognized that a single case of smallpox in the classroom could spread throughout an entire town. Consequently, in 1855, Massachusetts began requiring proof of smallpox vaccination for public school attendance. Parents opposed to vaccination could still send their children to private schools, and there were provisions for medical exemptions from the law. Other Massachusetts laws permitted local public health officials to require vaccination of individuals regardless of age if an outbreak of smallpox occurred. Those who refused could be fined $5 ($140 in 2018 dollars).

The Massachusetts approach to protecting public health by making sure school children were vaccinated became a model for other states. Today, all 50 states link public school attendance and proof of vaccination. In many states, the requirement extends to private schools, daycare facilities, and sometimes to enrollment into state colleges. All 50 states also allow physician-certified medical exemptions. All states except California, Mississippi, and West Virginia allow religious exemptions, and 17 states allow personal belief or philosophical exemptions.

Inevitably, the Massachusetts mandatory vaccination laws were challenged in court. In 1902, a smallpox epidemic developed in Cambridge, a small town outside of Boston, and local officials called for the vaccination of all residents. Most people cooperated, but a few resisted. One of those was Pastor Henning Jacobson. He claimed that he had been vaccinated in his native Sweden and had experienced lifelong pain and suffering as a result. When Cambridge officials ordered him to be vaccinated, he refused, and was fined. Instead of paying, he fought the fine in court. Although he was a pastor, his objection to vaccination was not based on religious beliefs. Instead, he argued that mandatory vaccination infringed on the liberty guaranteed him by the U.S. Constitution.

The case of *Jacobson v. Massachusetts* reached the U.S. Supreme Court in 1905. By that time, 11 states had enacted mandatory vaccination laws, so the case was of national interest. Jacobson lost his appeal by a 7–2 vote. Justice John Harlan delivered the majority opinion that concluded that

- mandatory vaccination was not inconsistent with protections guaranteed in the Fourteenth Amendment. The Amendment did not grant individuals the right to be free at all times of all personal restrictions;
- the state had the legal right to grant local health boards the power to enforce mandatory vaccination of all individuals during epidemics;
- individuals could be fined or jailed for refusing vaccination, but they could not be forcibly vaccinated against their wishes; and
- the law should not apply to any individual who could show that vaccination would impair health or cause death.

Jacobson v. Massachusetts became a foundation case for other legal challenges to mandatory vaccination. It established both the right of the state to require vaccination and the right to a personal health exemption. These principles continue to prevail today.

A new approach to invalidating compulsory vaccination laws arose in the case of *Zucht v. King*. It pitted the right to education against the school's requirement for proof of vaccination. In 1919, Rosalyn Zucht was not allowed to attend school in San Antonio, Texas, because she had no certificate of vaccination and refused to be vaccinated. The city had an ordinance that required any person attending either public or private school to show proof of vaccination. When she was excluded from school, Zucht filed suit. Her lawyers argued that

- the ordinance was unconstitutional because it gave the board of health the right to determine under what circumstances to enforce vaccination and thus under the Fourteenth Amendment deprived Rosalyn of her liberty without due process;
- the law deprived Rosalyn of her right to a free public education; and
- the law was discriminatory because it applied only to school children and not to others who might assemble in similar groups (e.g., adults at church).

In 1922, the U.S. Supreme Court refused to hear the Zucht case. It left in force a decision by a lower court that found the San Antonio ordinance was constitutional and that the board of health had the right to enforce the ordinance. The decision stated that the ordinance was not discriminatory and the right of a child to education did not take precedence over the right of the city to protect public health.

More recent lawsuits have concerned mandatory vaccination as a condition of employment. Courts generally have ruled that private employers such as hospitals and daycare centers can require employees to be vaccinated unless the vaccine will harm an individual's health. The most common employer-mandated vaccination is seasonal influenza.

PERSONAL CHOICE VIEW OF
MANDATORY VACCINATION

Personal choice advocates believe the government oversteps its authority by requiring healthy individuals to be vaccinated against their wishes. They believe parents should be free to decide for their children which vaccines to accept or reject, even though failure to vaccinate may spread a disease that results in the death of others. Although Jacobson's argument failed 100 years ago, personal choice advocates continue to claim the right to accept or reject vaccines as they see fit based on Section 1 of the Fourteenth Amendment to the U.S. Constitution, which reads:

> All persons born or naturalized in the United States, and subject to the jurisdiction thereof, are citizens of the United States and of the State wherein they reside. No State shall make or enforce any law which shall abridge the privileges or immunities of citizens of the United States; nor shall any State deprive any person of life, liberty, or property, without due process of law; nor deny to any person within its jurisdiction the equal protection of the laws.

These parents also insist that because mentally competent adults have the right to refuse medical treatment, and vaccination is a medical treatment, they should have the right to refuse vaccination for their children. They continue to fight in court to obtain what they consider to be their right.

On July 1, 2016, California Senate Bill 277 went into effect. It eliminated all personal belief vaccination exemptions which included religious exemptions. Medical exemptions certified by a physician were still permitted. A group of parents and the nonprofit organization Education 4 All filed suit in San Diego District Court to overturn the law. The basis for their suit was that the law was unconstitutionally discriminatory and that "SB 277 has made second class citizens out of children who for very compelling reasons are not vaccinated according to the CDC schedule" (Karlamangla, 2016). They asked that implementation of the law be delayed until its constitutionality could be determined. Their request was denied.

The International Chiropractors Association also quickly filed suit against SB 277 using the same argument as in *Zucht v. King* that mandatory vaccinations for all children except those with medical exemptions deprived children of the right to public education. Their request for delay was denied, and they withdrew the suit, stating that they would prepare a new lawsuit using different grounds to challenge the law. As of mid-2018, personal choice advocates in California have been unsuccessful in delaying or changing the law; however, since SB 277 was passed, no other states have changed their exemption policies.

Public Health View of Mandatory Vaccination

Public health officials see mandatory vaccination as the best way to protect citizens from contacting vaccine-preventable diseases. They point out that the courts have upheld compulsory vaccination laws for over a century. As mentioned earlier, some personal choice advocates insist that since mentally competent adults may legally refuse medical treatment and since vaccination is a medical treatment, parents should have the right to refuse vaccination for their children. However, courts have repeatedly rejected this argument on the basis that the government has a legitimate interest in child welfare. It can, for example, force parents to send their children to school, prevent them from sending young children to work, or remove them from their parents in cases of abuse and neglect. These precedents have been used to give states the legal right to compel vaccination of children against parental wishes.

In the view of public health officials, one of their responsibilities is to protect everyone in the community including people who cannot be vaccinated for medical reasons. Some people cannot receive a vaccine because they are taking drugs that suppress the immune system to prevent rejection of an organ transplant (see Case Study 5). Others have suppressed immune systems from receiving chemotherapy, while many more are living with immune-suppressing diseases such as HIV/AIDS. As medical treatments improve, people with weakened immune systems are living longer and their numbers are increasing, thus increasing the number of people who cannot be vaccinated and remain vulnerable to vaccine-preventable diseases.

The World Health Organization states that to be effective in stopping the spread of vaccine-preventable diseases, about 95 percent of the population must be vaccinated. When vaccination coverage reaches this level, herd immunity is created. With herd immunity, so few individuals are susceptible to a disease that there will be no large outbreak even if a few people still get sick. Those who cannot be vaccinated for medical reasons must depend on herd immunity to protect them from vaccine-preventable diseases, and it is the job of public health departments to see that these people are protected as much as possible. Public health officials believe the only way to achieve herd immunity and thus protect the medically unvaccinated is through mandatory vaccination laws.

Public health researchers have identified three distinct attitudes toward vaccination. There are vaccine acceptors, vaccine refusers, and those who are vaccine indifferent. The vaccine indifferent group has no strong feelings for or against vaccination, but because it is low on their list of concerns, they tend to vaccinate only if it is convenient or they are reminded to do so by others.

Children of the vaccine-indifferent group may not stay up-to-date with recommended vaccinations, not out of strong parental feelings but because of other barriers such as lack of accessible health care, difficulty with transportation, trouble scheduling convenient appointments, frequent relocation, language barriers, and everyday demands on parental time that push getting a child vaccinated low on their list of priorities. Laws that make vaccination mandatory for children to attend daycare or school push vaccine-indifferent parents to treat vaccinating as a higher priority by making it inconvenient for their children to remain unvaccinated. The California Department of Public Health reported that one school year after the state eliminated all but medical exemptions from vaccination, the percentage of kindergarteners statewide who had received all the CDC-recommended vaccines for their age rose from 92.9 percent to 95.6 percent. Both Los Angeles County and Orange County showed substantial 5 percent increases in fully vaccinated kindergarteners.

CHAPTER 13

Is Negative Information about Vaccines Suppressed?

The idea that governments and the pharmaceutical industry cover up or distort negative information about vaccines is nothing new. For example, between 1955 and 1963, some batches of rhesus monkey kidney cells used in making polio vaccine were contaminated with a monkey virus called SV40. Questions developed about whether SV40 increased the risk of developing certain cancers. The Institute of Medicine (IOM) investigated, but because there was no way to determine which people were given the contaminated vaccine, the IOM did not come to a definitive conclusion. Anti-vaccinationists claimed that health officials suppressed results that would have clearly linked the vaccine to cancer.

In 1992, journalist Tom Curtis published a story in *Rolling Stone* magazine loosely connecting a series of events that he claimed showed a polio vaccine was responsible for the spread of AIDS. Hilary Koprowski, a vaccine researcher, developed a live polio vaccine that was used from 1957 to 1960 in parts of Africa where HIV/AIDS was emerging. Koprowski sued *Rolling Stone* for defamation, and the magazine was forced to admit the article was not based on any scientific research. It published a statement clearing Dr. Koprowski and the vaccine from any association with AIDS.

This statement simply reinforced the belief of anti-vaccinationists that the press and the government were suppressing information that would prove a polio vaccine–AIDS connection. Seven years later, British journalist Edward Hooper published *The River: A Journey to the Source of HIV and AIDS*. The book claimed a polio vaccine–AIDS link and suppression of this information, even though many researchers could find no connection. Despite this, as of 2018, Hooper continued to promote the story on his website.

The idea of the government conspiring with the pharmaceutical indus-try to suppress information about vaccine–disease links refuses to die. The problem is not just an American one. In certain areas of Nigeria in 2017, tribal leaders told parents not to vaccinate their children against polio because vaccination was a secret government plot to sterilize Muslim girls.

Researchers have tried to understand why vaccine conspiracy theories have such a vigorous life. One trend is a growing distrust in the trans-parency of government agencies and large corporations, especially phar-maceutical manufacturers. The megaphone of social media amplifies this trend. By one estimate, in 2017, anti-vaccine conspiracy theorists had more than seven million followers on Facebook alone. This does not include all the readers of anti-vaccination websites and blogs of self-identified anti-vaccine experts. As many as 80 percent of people search for health-related information on the internet. When looking for vaccine information, they are likely to come across sites that promote conspiracy theories. These may reinforce already held beliefs and play on their fears as parents, mak-ing it difficult to counter incorrect information.

ANTI-VACCINATIONIST VIEW ON SUPPRESSION OF INFORMATION

"We all know by now that our 'free press' has deeply embedded editors and producers who take their marching orders directly from pharmaceuti-cal companies and the CDC. Their job is to postpone, water down, spin, or kill stories that hurt public health profits," writes an anti-vaccination blog-ger who writes under the name Levi Quackenboss (Quackenboss, 2017). This is an extreme but common view among anti-vaccination conspir-acy theorists. They believe any positive information on vaccines coming from the government or vaccine makers is suspicious and false and that all negative data on vaccines are covered up or censored.

Richard Jaffee, the attorney who defended vaccine-skeptic Dr. Robert Sears who was brought up on charges before the California Medical Board (see Chapter 12), makes similar claims as Quackenboss, only in less inflammatory language. "I keep hearing the same thing over and over again," he writes. "The academic expert is concerned about vaccine safety but can't go public because of fear of reprisals from the vaccine Mafioso" (Jaffee, 2017).

Some vaccine conspiracy theorists blame profit motives of pharmaceu-tical companies for covering up data they are convinced show vaccines are unsafe. These anti-vaccinationists also claim the industry develops and knowingly pushes unnecessary vaccines and unneeded booster shots to increase profits and that the government and mainstream press are complicit in helping the industry fool the public into thinking that vaccines are safe and effective.

Other anti-vaccinationists claim the government knows vaccines are unsafe but that it has joined a conspiracy to cover up this information because if it became public, the government would be liable for millions of dollars in damages. For example, anti-vaccine activist Robert Kennedy, Jr., claimed in an article published in *Rolling Stone* and Salon.com in 2005 that in 2000 a group of top officials from the Centers for Disease Control and Prevention (CDC), the Food and Drug Administration, the World Health Organization, and vaccine manufacturers held a top-secret meeting in Norcross, Georgia, specifically to suppress information that thimerosal in vaccines causes autism, a connection that has been conclusively exposed as false (see Chapter 10).

The 2016 movie *Vaxxed: From Cover-up to Catastrophe,* written and directed by Andrew Wakefield (see Chapter 10) claimed to show another government conspiracy. It charged that the CDC covered up and destroyed data that proved a link between the MMR vaccine and autism. The movie quoted William Thompson, a senior scientist at the CDC, to support its point. Thompson later claimed his comments were inappropriately edited (see below).

Constant repetition that the government and pharmaceutical industry cannot be trusted has depressed vaccination rates and influenced ordinary people. The 2018 influenza outbreak was one of the worst in recent years. In the Lehigh Valley in Pennsylvania, so many people went to the emergency rooms with flu symptoms that one hospital set up a triage tent in the parking lot to accommodate them. After being sick for five days, 22-year-old Sarah Rogers arrived at this tent. When asked if she had gotten a flu shot, she said no, because she had heard that the flu shot gives you flu and "you can get Alzheimer's from it—that there's mercury in it, and it goes to your brain" (McNeil, 2018). When asked from where she had gotten that idea, which is contradictory to all research findings, she said she had learned these "facts" on social media.

MAINSTREAM MEDICAL VIEW ON INFORMATION SUPPRESSION

Vaccine researchers and mainstream physicians believe that observation, controlled testing, analysis, and repetition of the process by multiple independent researchers produce accurate, reproducible, truthful information that can be applied to improve public health. Scientists all over the

world work on developing and testing vaccines and then objectively ana-
lyze the data from their work. They submit their results to peer-reviewed
journals for other scientists to evaluate, and their published information is
available to other scientists, journalists, and the public. To suppress, cover
up, or destroy negative evidence about vaccines would require a worldwide conspiracy involving dozens of countries and thousands of people.

Pharmaceutical companies are in business to make a profit for their
shareholders, but vaccines are not a big profit center for the industry,
regardless of what anti-vaccinationists think. In 2016, it took on average
$2.6 billion to bring a new drug to market. New vaccines tend to be even
more costly because of the length of time it takes to develop and test them
and the need to build new, specialized facilities to produce them. In 2016,
the global pharmaceutical market was worth $1.05 trillion. Vaccines were
between 2 percent and 3 percent of this market and produced only a small
profit compared to other classes of drugs.

As for the Robert Kennedy, Jr.'s claims that the government held a
conference at the Simpsonwood Retreat in Norcross, Georgia, to cover
up a link between thimerosal and autism, the U.S. Senate Committee on
Health, Education, Labor, and Pensions investigated the allegations. The
committee's conclusion was that "Allegations of a cover-up are not sub-
stantiated . . . Instead of hiding the data or restricting access to it, CDC distributed it, often to individuals who had never seen it before, and solicited
outside opinion regarding how to interpret it. The transcript of these dis-
cussions was made available to the public" (U.S. Senate, 2007, 6). Salon.
com retracted Kennedy's article because of major factual errors.

The movie *Vaxxed: From Cover-up to Catastrophe* claims that scientists
at the CDC covered up and destroyed evidence about a study that showed
a connection between MMR vaccine and autism. This claim is based on
telephone conversations between William Thompson, a senior scientist
at the CDC, and anti-vaccinationist Brian Hooker. Thompson expressed
concern that a subset of experimental data suggested that African American
boys who received the MMR vaccine before age three years were at
increased risk of autism. This data had been omitted from an article
published in the journal *Pediatrics*. Thompson viewed this omission as
a failure to follow the study protocol. When challenged, the CDC said the
data were omitted because the apparent correlation did not hold up under
a more in-depth statistical analysis.

Unknown to Thompson and without his permission, Hooker recorded
their calls. Parts of the recorded calls were pieced together in *Vaxxed* in
such a way as to suggest a deliberate cover-up at the CDC and to promote
the Wakefield theory that MMR vaccine causes autism. After the film was

released, Thompson retained a law firm to represent him and through the law firm issued this statement: "I believe vaccines have saved and continue to save countless lives. I would never suggest that any parent avoid vaccinating children of any race. Vaccines prevent serious diseases, and the risks associated with their administration are vastly outweighed by their individual and societal benefits" (Thompson, 2014).

Why people hold so firmly to the belief that negative information about vaccines is being covered up or destroyed confounds the medical establishment. An article published in 2018 in the American Psychological Association journal *Health Psychology* attempted to identify the type of person who believes negative vaccine data were being suppressed. The researchers surveyed more than 5,000 people in 24 countries. They found that people who believed other conspiracy theories such as that Princess Diana was murdered or that the U.S. government knew in advance about the 2001 attack on New York's World Trade Center and allowed the attack to happen were more likely to hold anti-vaccination and vaccine conspiracy views. This correlation existed independent of nationality or education level.

The mainstream medical establishment would dismiss claims that the government, pharmaceutical industry, and press work together to cover up negative information about vaccines as completely ridiculous except that this theory has spread through social media and lowered vaccination rates. The medical establishment has found conspiracy theories about suppression of negative vaccine data, although wildly untrue, are very difficult to eliminate. So long as these theories continue to circulate on the internet, they will put children's lives at unnecessary risk.

PART III

Scenarios

Case Studies

CASE STUDY 1: ALLISON IS HOMESCHOOLED

In March 2016, Allison was a sixth grader in a Marin, California, public school. She was a good student and looked forward to going to junior high with her friends Divya and Sami. Toward the end of the year, the school sent home paperwork with all sixth graders explaining the procedure for parents to enroll their children in junior high school. Allison took the information home, gave it to her mother, Rebecca, and did not think any more about it.

A few days later, Rebecca looked at the information and came across a paragraph concerning health information and sports physicals for entering seventh graders. Included was a reminder that state law now required all entering seventh graders to have proof of vaccination against diphtheria, pertussis, tetanus, mumps, measles, and rubella. The only way to obtain an exception from this requirement was to have written waiver from a licensed physician. The waiver had to include a statement saying

- the child has a specific medical condition that prevents safe immunization;
- the vaccines the child is exempt from receiving; and
- whether the exemption is temporary or permanent, and if temporary, when the exemption expires.

Rebecca was angry at what she considered intrusion of the government into a decision she thought was her right to make as a parent. Allison had never been vaccinated. Rebecca had read on the internet that vaccines were both risky and ineffective. Her pediatrician had been sympathetic to Rebecca's concerns, and although she had encouraged Rebecca to vaccinate Allison, she had not insisted when Rebecca stated her firm objections.

There was no way Rebecca would expose her precious daughter to this unnecessary medical procedure. She called a friend who was a vaccine skeptic for advice on how to avoid the requirement.

"This is ridiculous," she told the friend. "Who gets diphtheria these days? How many people do you know who have had measles or mumps?"

"Call your pediatrician and see if she will write an exemption for Allison," the friend suggested.

Rebecca called her pediatrician and asked for a medical exemption, but the doctor refused. She said nothing in Allison's medical records indicated there was any reason Allison could not be vaccinated.

"I have to follow the law," the doctor said. "Besides, I know you are concerned, but there are good reasons to vaccinate, and the chance of any problems are tiny—less than one in a million."

After the doctor turned down Rebecca's request for a medical exemption, Rebecca went on the internet looking for a solution. She discovered that homeschooled children do not have to be vaccinated. Soon she connected online with a group of Marin homeschoolers and made the decision that she would homeschool Allison rather than allow her to receive the required vaccines.

August arrived. Divya and Sami were excited about going to junior high. Allison seemed sullen and would not talk about school.

"Let's all go to orientation together," Sami suggested.

"I'm not going," Allison said. "My mom says those shots the school says I have to have are not safe. She's going to homeschool me. She doesn't care that I want to get the shots, so I can go to school and be with my friends."

"That's mean," said Divya. "I had to have a bunch of shots when my family moved here from India. They made my arm sore for a couple of days, but they didn't make me sick or anything."

Despite Allison's insistence that she wanted to go to junior high like her friends, Rebecca followed through on homeschooling. Allison missed Divya and Sami and the excitement of starting a new school year. At first, the three friends saw each other on weekends, but as Divya and Sami got involved in school life, they had less and less in common with Allison, and they gradually drifted apart. Allison eventually made a new friend in the homeschooling group, but whenever she was mad at her mother, she brought up how unfair it was that Rebecca would not let her be vaccinated and go to regular school.

Analysis

Rebecca clearly held strong negative beliefs about vaccination. Until January 1, 2016, parents in California could exempt their child from any or all school-required vaccinations if vaccination was contrary to their personal beliefs. To do this, a parent had to fill out a form and discuss the risks and benefits of immunizations with a health care practitioner. The form needed to be filed twice, once before the child entered kindergarten and again before the child entered seventh grade. Before Allison entered kindergarten, Rebecca had filed a personal belief exemption statement that allowed Allison to attend school through sixth grade while avoiding vaccination.

California Senate Bill 277 (SB277) was signed into law in June 2015 and became effective on January 1, 2016. This bill eliminated all personal belief exemptions from vaccination. Unlike many states, California had no separate religious belief exemption; so, once the law became effective, the only permitted exemptions were for medical reasons confirmed by a medical or osteopathic doctor. Rebecca could no longer exempt Allison from vaccination based on her own belief that they were harmful, and Allison's pediatrician was following the law in refusing to write a medical exemption for her when she had no medical condition preventing vaccination.

Vaccination is a condition of public school entry everywhere in the United States and private school entry in most states, including California. However, fully homeschooled children are not required to be vaccinated. Rebecca's opposition to vaccination was so firm that she chose to withdraw Allison from the public school system. Allison remained healthy despite her vulnerability to vaccine-preventable diseases. Rebecca's decision may or may not have affected the quality of Allison's education, but it had the unintended consequence of affecting her social relationships with her former classmates at a time when peer relationships become of increasing importance, something Allison continued to resent.

CASE STUDY 2: DANIEL GETS ROTAVIRUS

Roger and Bethany Peterson were thrilled when their first child, Daniel, was born a healthy 7.5 lb. (2.8 kg) boy. They were surprised when the morning before he was to be discharged from the hospital, a nurse announced that it was time for Daniel to have his hepatitis B shot.

"Wait a minute," Roger said. "What's this shot all about?"

"It's a vaccine against the liver disease hepatitis B," the nurse explained. "It's recommended for all newborns."

"I've never heard of babies getting hepatitis B," Bethany said. "How common is it?"

"It's usually a sexually transmitted disease," the nurse said. "The vaccine now will make sure your child never gets infected."

"You're telling me you're giving this two-day-old baby a shot for something he won't be exposed to for years?"

"It's the best way to protect him," the nurse said.

"No." said Roger. "No shot. He's too young. He can get it when he is older." Bethany nodded in agreement, and Daniel went home without getting the hepatitis B vaccine.

At his two-month checkup, Daniel was scheduled to receive the first dose of five vaccines: diphtheria, tetanus, and pertussis (DTaP); inactivated polio (IPV); rotavirus; *Haemophilus influenzae* type b; and pneumococcal conjugate (PCV13).

"That's a lot of vaccines all at once," Bethany said. "How do I know he won't have a bad reaction?"

The nurse explained the diseases each shot prevented and how serious they could be for an infant. The doctor also talked to Bethany about how safe the vaccines were and how giving so many together did not increase the risk unwanted reactions. Bethany was skeptical. In the end, she refused the IPV and rotavirus vaccines for her son.

A few weeks later, Daniel developed a fever and began vomiting and producing frequent watery diarrhea. Bethany felt like she was changing his diaper every hour. At first, Daniel cried and fussed, but after half a day, he became quiet and limp and was not interested in nursing. This frightened Bethany more than his crying. When Roger came home from work, they decided to take Daniel to the urgent care center.

The doctor at the urgent care center was concerned that Daniel was extremely dehydrated and unresponsive, so he sent the couple to the hospital emergency room. The ER doctor put Daniel on an intravenous drip to restore his fluids and asked the couple if Daniel had been vaccinated against rotavirus.

Bethany said she had refused that vaccine. The doctor frowned and said rotavirus was likely the cause of the fever, diarrhea, and dehydration. He decided Daniel should stay overnight in the hospital for observation. Roger was annoyed at Bethany for not letting the pediatrician give Daniel all the recommended vaccines, and Bethany felt guilty that her son was now sick enough to be hospitalized.

Daniel returned home the next day and recovered without complications from his bout with rotavirus. Bethany and Roger had been frightened by how quickly Daniel had gone from being a healthy baby to being seriously ill. They agreed that, from now on, they would accept the vaccine recommendations of the pediatrician.

Analysis

Many parents like Bethany and Roger are concerned about their child getting so many vaccines at such a young age. Although Daniel was highly unlikely to encounter hepatitis B as an infant, the recommendation that he receive the vaccine before leaving the hospital was a public health measure. If all children are vaccinated at birth, it may be possible to eliminate the disease. However, if Daniel receives the vaccine at an older age but before he becomes sexually active, it can be equally effective.

Combination vaccines and giving multiple shots at a single office visit are also a concern for some parents because they believe that the baby's immune system may be unable to handle the number of antigens present in multiple shots. The development of subunit vaccines, which use only a few proteins from a virus or bacterium instead of the entire organism to stimulate immunity, has substantially reduced the number of antigens in vaccines. Between 1980 and 2016, the number of antigens in vaccines given to children under one year old has been reduced from over 3,000 to just over 150, even though the child receives more vaccines against more diseases in 2016 than in 1980.

The recommended immunization schedule takes into consideration the maturity of the baby's immune system and the age at which a child is most vulnerable to each disease. Rotavirus vaccine is given only to children under six months old because the first year of life is when they are most vulnerable to fatal dehydration. Before a rotavirus vaccine was available, the virus was responsible for between 2 million and 3 million cases of diarrhea and 70,000 hospitalizations every year in the United States. In 2018, it is still the leading cause of dehydration in children worldwide, causing about 125 million cases of diarrhea and more than 500,000 deaths each year.

Hib vaccine, which protects against a bacterial infection caused by *Haemophilus influenzae* type b, and DTaP, which protects against diphtheria, tetanus, and pertussis (whooping cough), are also recommended at two months because these diseases are most serious and potentially fatal in young children. Both the *Haemophilus influenzae* bacterium and the pertussis bacterium can be spread by carriers who do not always show symptoms of the disease. By delaying these immunizations, parents leave their children vulnerable to diseases at a time when they are most likely to cause serious complications.

Case Study 3: Miguel Has Chickenpox as an Adult

Miguel is 30 years old and was born in Arizona. In 1994, when he was six, his mother got a new job that it required her to be away from home for long periods, so Miguel went to live with his grandparents in Mexico. Up to that point, Miguel had had all the recommended childhood vaccinations. Miguel lived with his grandparents for three years.

In 1995, when the varicella vaccine against chicken pox was licensed in the United States, Miguel was living in Mexico, so he did not receive the vaccine. When his mother's job changed, and he returned to live with her in Arizona, school officials asked his mother if he had already had chickenpox. She was not sure, but she knew he had been sick with a rash when living with his grandparents, so she said yes. At that time, a parent's word that his or her child had contracted chickenpox was all the school required for the child to enroll, although today written proof is required. In junior high school, Miguel once again lived for an extended period with his grandparents, but no one in either country ever asked about whether he had been vaccinated against chickenpox or had the disease.

Miguel graduated from high school and went to college. In his junior year during spring break, he traveled with a youth group from his college to help earthquake victims in Mexico City. On the last day of his stay, he began to feel achy and feverish. By the time he got back to his dorm room, he noticed that he had a few red spots on his face. The next morning, the rash covered much of his face and chest, and he felt uncomfortably itchy, had a high fever, and experienced spells of dizziness that scared him. At the university health center, the doctor told him he had chickenpox and isolated him in the health center infirmary.

"I thought chickenpox was a disease kids got," Miguel said.

"Most kids now get vaccinated against the disease, so it is much less common than it used to be," the doctor said. "Adults who get it were never vaccinated and never had chickenpox as a kid. For kids, it's usually a mild disease, but adults get much sicker and take longer to get over it."

Miguel remained isolated and contagious for 10 days until his chickenpox blisters slowly scabbed over. He missed two weeks of classes and had to struggle to catch up but was fortunate to recover without any of the serious complications that often occur in adults.

Analysis

Miguel left the United States before the varicella vaccine was available. After that, moving between the United States and Mexico, he fell through the health care cracks and was never vaccinated. At the time he entered school in the United States, vaccination requirements were loosely enforced in Arizona, and a parent's statement that a child had already contracted chickenpox was adequate for school admission until 2011.

Mexico and the United States have different immunization recommendations. For example, varicella vaccine is recommended in Mexico only for high-risk groups, while it is recommended for all children in the United States. Today the CDC issues a binational immunization resource tool designed specifically to address vaccination coverage for children who move between Mexico and the United States. The tool helps families to fully meet the school entry requirements of both countries.

As Miguel found out, some normally mild vaccine-preventable childhood diseases such as chickenpox are much more serious in adults. It often takes adults two to three weeks to recover even without complications. Complications from adult chickenpox can include pneumonia, and bone, joint, and brain infections.

Adults like Miguel, who may not know if they ever have had chickenpox or another vaccine-preventable disease or who are unsure if they have been vaccinated against them, can have a blood test to determine if they have made antibodies against the disease. People of all ages who apply for permanent residency in the United States are required by federal law to prove they have had all the CDC-recommended vaccines for their age. This is the only federal immunization requirement. All other immunization requirements are regulated by individual states and generally apply only to school entry.

Case Study 4: Ella Has Seizures

Dwayne and Maggie Richards were thrilled when after several failed attempts to adopt a baby they were able to bring home six-month-old Ella from China. They had received very limited information about Ella from the agency that had arranged the adoption and even less from the orphanage where she had lived since she was a few weeks old. On arriving back in the United States, their priority was to get Ella thoroughly checked by a pediatrician they had preselected.

The pediatrician examined Ella and found she was healthy although small for her age. Since Dwayne and Maggie had no idea if Ella had received any immunizations, the pediatrician started her on a catch-up vaccination schedule. Ella tolerated the shots well with no unexpected reactions or complications. By the time she was one year old, her immunizations were up-to-date. At 15 months, she received the combined mumps, measles, and rubella (MMR) vaccine. A few days later, she cried for hours and had a fever of 40°C (104°F).

Maggie was holding Ella trying to calm her when Ella's eyes rolled back in her head. Her body stiffened and she began twitching. Dwayne and Maggie were horrified. Convinced that Ella was dying, they rushed her to the emergency room. On the way there, she experienced another seizure, but once they reached the hospital, she seemed normal but limp and exhausted.

The emergency room doctor reviewed Ella's health history and explained that Ella had experienced febrile seizures brought on by her high fever. He assured the Richards that these seizures were fairly common in young children. Since Ella had no other signs of illness, he suggested the fever might be related to her recent MMR shot, but cautioned that there was no way to know for sure whether the shot had caused the fever. After taking steps to bring Ella's temperature down, she was discharged with instructions to take her to her pediatrician for follow-up tests to make sure the seizures did not indicate a serious problem.

The next day Ella still had a fever, but it was lower, and she seemed more like herself. Her pediatrician reassured the Richards that although febrile seizures were frightening, they caused no lasting damage. He scheduled some additional tests for Ella, and the results showed no signs of epilepsy or any other seizure disorder.

Ella continued to grow into a healthy child, experiencing only normal, transient childhood illnesses. When she was four, Maggie took her for her well child checkup where she was scheduled to receive her second MMR shot. Although Maggie believed in vaccinating, she wanted to be careful not to do anything that could harm Ella. At the appointment, she reminded the doctor of the seizure episode.

"Are you sure Ella isn't going to have more seizures with this second MMR shot?" Maggie asked.

"I think it unlikely," the pediatrician said, "but I can't guarantee that she won't."

"Then I don't want her to have the shot," Maggie said. "Since she is adopted, we don't know anything about her family medical history or whether she might be allergic to something in the shot."

"I strongly recommend a second MMR shot," the doctor said. "Odds are she will be just fine, but we don't have to immunize her today. Go home and think about it."

Maggie went home and talked the situation over with Dwayne. They learned that between 95 percent and 98 percent of people develop immunity to measles with only one shot. Based on that information, they decided to skip the second MMR vaccination.

Analysis

Five to fifteen percent of children who develop a fever after the MMR shot have a temperature of 103°F (39.4°C) or higher, five to twelve days after vaccination. The fever lasts one to two days and can cause seizures. Febrile seizures, although they do not cause any lasting harm, are frightening for parents. Dwayne and Maggie were at a disadvantage because they knew nothing about Ella's family or health history. After the emergency room doctor suggested that Ella's fever could be the result of her recent MMR shot, they did some reading about the MMR vaccine on the CDC website and decided to be cautious and have Ella skip the second shot.

Dwayne and Maggie were comfortable with this decision because they had learned that most people make enough antibodies from a single MMR shot to protect them against measles. They understood that a single dose of MMR vaccine was less effective against mumps and rubella, but decided these diseases were less serious than measles, and the risk that Ella would contract them was low.

One alternative Dwayne and Maggie did not consider was having Ella tested to see if she had made adequate antibodies against measles, mumps, and rubella from the first shot. This can be done with a simple blood antigen test. Some selective vaccinators also use this approach. They delay giving their child MMR, varicella, and hepatitis A vaccines, and, when the child is about 11 years old, have a blood test done to see if the child has acquired natural immunity to any of these diseases. If not, they may choose to vaccinate because symptoms and complications of these diseases in teens and adults are usually much more serious than in children.

As a precaution, because Ella has no way of knowing if she is protected against rubella, she should have an antigen test as an adult before trying to become pregnant. Rubella in the mother during pregnancy can cause serious birth defects in the developing baby. Should Ella not have enough antibodies to protect her against rubella, she should have another MMR shot as an adult and wait at least a month before trying to conceive.

CASE STUDY 5: CHARLIE CANNOT BE VACCINATED

Charlie was diagnosed with acute lymphocytic leukemia (ALL) when he was four years old. Leukemias are cancers of the blood. ALL is the most common type of childhood cancer. With ALL, the cells in the bone marrow mature into abnormal, cancerous blood cells rather than healthy blood cells.

Charlie was treated at a special children's cancer center, but his initial treatment was not successful. Eventually, his doctors decided that his best chance of beating the cancer was a stem cell transplant. To prepare for the procedure, Charlie received heavy doses of chemotherapy that left him weak and nauseated. The chemotherapy was necessary to kill all the blood-producing cells in his bone marrow, but it also killed a lot of healthy immune system cells. This left Charlie with little protection against infection.

The stem cell transplant worked. The stem cells settled in Charlie's bone marrow where they reproduced and matured into healthy blood cells. The recovery period was long, and Charlie and his family had to take extra precautions to make sure he did not contract any infectious diseases because his immune system was still weak. In addition, Charlie could not be immunized with any vaccine that contained a live attenuated (weakened) virus. The possibility existed that even a weakened live virus in the vaccine could overwhelm his fragile immune system. This meant that he received a medical exemption from the varicella and MMR vaccines.

When Charlie was seven, he was finally healthy enough to attend school. He still could not be given varicella or MMR vaccine, and if he caught any of these diseases, his symptoms and complications would be much more serious, and possibly life-threatening, than they would be if a healthy but unvaccinated child got sick.

Before enrolling Charlie in public school, his parents went to the school and explained his health situation and their concern about his exposure to vaccine-preventable diseases. They asked the school to assure them that the other pupils were all vaccinated to protect Charlie's health. The school's response was that it could not accommodate that request. The state Charlie lived in allowed both medical and religious exemptions. The school could not force parents with religious exemptions to vaccinate. In addition, health privacy laws prohibited them from telling Charlie's parents which children were not vaccinated or separating vaccinated and unvaccinated children into separate classrooms.

Charlie's parents were frustrated and angry that the school would not help them. They had been through a lot, both financially and emotionally, during Charlie's cancer treatment. To them, the request seemed logical and necessary. When it became clear that their request would be denied, they decided to sue the school for failing to provide a safe environment for Charlie. While the case worked its way through the courts, the school system offered Charlie homebound instruction. The school district paid for a tutor to go to Charlie's house several times each week with assignments and to monitor his progress. Although this met Charlie academic needs, it did not meet his social need, while the legal case remained unresolved.

Analysis

In this situation, the right of parents to exempt their children from vaccination for religious reasons, health privacy laws, and the right of a special needs child to a free public education conflict. Once children like Charlie are healthy enough, doctors generally recommend that they attend regular school for both psychological, social, and academic reasons. Schools, however, feel their ability to accommodate some families' requests is limited.

Since Charlie is medically exempt from certain vaccinations, his family wants him to be protected from the transmission of vaccine-preventable diseases by herd immunity. To do this, the vaccine status of each classmate must be reviewed, and parents of unvaccinated children must be forced to vaccinate. In a state with religious or personal belief exemptions from vaccination, that is not legally possible.

Several lawsuits like Charlie's have been filed in various states, but there has been no clear resolution of the conflicting rights. One possible solution is for other states to pass laws like those in Mississippi, West Virginia, and California, which eliminate religious and personal belief exemptions. So long as these nonexemption laws are rigorously enforced, children with medical exemptions from vaccination are then protected at school by herd immunity and no health privacy laws are broken.

TIMELINE

1549 The first written record of variolation against smallpox appears in Chinese literature.

1721 Lady Mary Wortley Montagu introduces variolation to England.

1721 Violent opposition to variolation occurs in Boston during a smallpox epidemic.

1777 General George Washington begins mandatory variolation of soldiers in the Continental Army.

1796 British doctor Edward Jenner develops smallpox vaccine using cowpox virus.

1840 The British Vaccination Act of 1840 makes variolation illegal and provides free cowpox vaccinations for the poor.

1853 The Vaccine Act of 1853 makes smallpox infant vaccination mandatory in England and Wales, the first British attempt at legislating compulsory vaccination.

1854 The British Anti-Vaccination League is formed to protest the Vaccine Act.

1855 Massachusetts becomes the first state to require smallpox vaccination for public school attendance.

1867 The British Anti-Compulsory Vaccination League is founded in response to the new law that requires all children under age 14 be vaccinated.

1871 Parliament mandates that British mandatory vaccination laws be vigorously enforced with increased punishments for noncompliance.

1879 The Anti-Vaccination Society of America is founded.

1882 The New England Anti-Compulsory Vaccination League is founded.

1885 The Anti-Vaccination League of New York City is founded.

1885 Tens of thousands attend the Leicester Demonstration March against vaccination in England.

1898 British Parliament passes the Vaccination Act of 1898, allowing conscientious objections and dropping fines for noncompliance. This ends Britain's first attempt at mandatory vaccination.

1902 Vaccine resister Henning Jacobson goes to court to challenge Massachusetts's vaccination laws. He loses the case and appeals to the U.S. Supreme Court.

1902 U.S. Congress passes the Biologics Control Act, requiring manufactures of antitoxins, serums, and vaccines to be inspected and licensed annually.

1905 *Jacobson v. Massachusetts* is decided by the Supreme Court in favor of the state, establishing the legality of mandatory vaccination but permitting medical exemptions.

1906 U.S. Congress passes the Pure Food and Drug Act that prohibits the manufacture, sale, or transportation of all adulterated, mislabeled, or poisonous foods, drugs, and medicines.

1919 Rosalyn Zucht goes to court to challenge school vaccination laws in San Antonio, Texas. She loses the case and appeals to the Supreme Court.

1922 The Supreme Court refuses to hear *Zucht v. King* and leaves standing a lower court decision that San Antonio's laws are legal and do not conflict with the right to a free public education.

1955 Jonas Salk's polio vaccine is licensed in the United States.

1972 United States stops routine vaccination against smallpox.

1974 The Association of Parents of Vaccine Damaged Children is founded in England.

1979 The last case of native polio occurs in the United States.

1980 Smallpox is declared eradicated.

1982 *DPT: Vaccine Roulette* is aired on television, marking the beginning of the modern anti-vaccination movement.

1982 Dissatisfied Parents Together (now called the National Vaccine Information Center) is founded to demand government recognition of vaccine dangers.

1986 The National Childhood Vaccine Injury Act creates the National Vaccine Program Office to coordinate all federal government immunization-related activities.

1988 The Vaccine Injury Compensation Program begins operating.

1990 The Vaccine Adverse Event Reporting System is created.

1998 British doctor Andrew Wakefield announces his research shows (falsely) that the MMR vaccine is associated with the development of autism.

2000 U.S. Congressman Dan Burton holds hearings on mercury in vaccines.

2000 Native measles is eliminated in the United States. Imported cases still occur.

2001 Manufacturers stop using thimerosal in vaccines in the United States for children under age six years except for influenza vaccine.

2016 A California law goes into effect, making it the third state to allow only documented medical exemptions from vaccination.

2016 The International Chiropractors Association files suit against the California vaccination law, but later withdraws the suit.

2017 Italy changes its vaccination laws to allow only medical exemptions after a widespread outbreak of measles.

2018 France makes 11 vaccinations mandatory for children born after January 1, 2018, in response to increases in cases of vaccine-preventable diseases.

2018 The British Veterinary Association issues a statement that dogs do not get autism in response to anti-vaccine rumors that canine vaccines can cause autism in dogs.

SOURCES FOR FURTHER INFORMATION

PRO-VACCINE RESOURCES

Bill & Melinda Gates Foundation
440 5th Ave North
Seattle, WA 98109
206-709-3100
https://www.gatesfoundation.org
The Gates Foundation is a philanthropic organization with substantial interest in eradicating polio, malaria, and HIV infection. The organization supports the Decade of Vaccines Global Vaccine Action Plan that aims to provide universal vaccination by 2020.

Center for Biologics Evaluation and Research
10001 New Hampshire Avenue
Silver Spring, MD 20993-0002
800-835-4709 (toll free); 240-402-8010 (local)
ocod@fda.hhs.gov
https://www.fda.gov/AboutFDA/CentersOffices/OfficeofMedical-ProductsandTobacco/CBER/default.htm
A division of the Food and Drug Administration, the Center for Biologics Evaluation and Research is responsible for ensuring the safety, purity, potency, and effectiveness of biological products, including vaccines, blood and blood products, and cells, tissues, and gene therapies. This includes the approval, compliance, and surveillance of vaccines. Information is available in 16 languages.

Children's Hospital of Philadelphia Vaccine Education Center
3 401 Civic Center Blvd.
Philadelphia, PA 19104
800-879-2467
https://www.chop.edu/centers-programs/vaccine-education-center
The Vaccine Education Center serves as a resource for parents with questions about the safety and effectiveness of vaccination.

The College of Physicians of Philadelphia
19 South 22nd Street
Philadelphia, PA 19103-3097
215-399-2253
https://www.historyofvaccines.org
This organization maintains a website documenting the history of vaccines and discussing some of the controversies surrounding them.

Gavi, the Vaccine Alliance
1776 I Street, NW, Suite 600
Washington, DC 20006
202-478-1050
https://www.gavi.org
Created in 2000, this international organization brings together public and private organizations involved in providing access to new and underused vaccines for children in underserved areas.

Immunization Action Coalition
2550 University Avenue West, Suite 415 North
Saint Paul, MN 55114
651-647-9009
admin@immunize.org
http://www.immunize.org and http://www.vaccineinformation.org
A pro-vaccination organization that is funded in part by the U.S. Centers for Disease Control and Prevention to educate health care professionals and the public about U.S. vaccine recommendations.

Institute for Vaccine Safety
Johns Hopkins Bloomberg School of Public Health
615 N. Wolfe Street, Room W5041
Baltimore, MD 21205
410-955-3543
info@hopkinsvaccine.org

http://www.vaccinesafety.edu
Established in 1992 at Johns Hopkins University, this organization strives to provide an independent assessment of vaccines and vaccine safety to help educate decision makers, physicians, the public, and the media about issues of vaccine safety in the interest of preventing disease using the safest vaccines possible.

National Foundation for Infectious Diseases
7201 Wisconsin Avenue, Suite 750
Bethesda, MD 20814
301-656-0003
https://www.nfid.org
This organization supports U.S. vaccination policy by providing education and vaccine resources for daycares, schools, and workplaces. The site also includes links to vaccine education lesson plans for teachers.

Public Health Agency of Canada
130 Colonnade Road, A.L. 6501H
Ottawa, Ontario K1A 0K9
844-280-5020 (toll free in Canada)
https://www.publichealth.gc.ca
This gateway site is sponsored by the government of Canada for citizens to access information on infectious diseases, immunization, travel health, and other health issues. Text is available in English and French.

U.S. Centers for Disease Control and Prevention (CDC)
600 Clifton Road
Atlanta, GA 30329-4027
800-CDC-INFO (toll free); 888-232-6348 (for hearing impaired)
https://www.cdc.gov
The CDC is a government organization that is part of the Department of Health and Human Services. Its mission is to educate and protect the health of Americans. The site provides official information on every vaccine as well recommended vaccine schedules and travel vaccination requirements. Text is available in 16 languages.

U.S. Court of Federal Claims/Vaccine Claims
Howard T. Markey National Courts Building
717 Madison Place, NW

Washington, DC 20439
202-357-6400
http://www.uscfc.uscourts.gov/vaccine-programoffice-special-masters
This court was established to hear claims of injury under the National
Vaccine Injury Compensation Program and the National Childhood
Vaccine Injury Act of 1986. The website explains how the program
works and how to file a claim.

U.S. Food and Drug Administration (FDA)
10903 New Hampshire Avenue
Silver Spring, MD 20993
888-463-6332 (toll free)
https://www.fda.gov
This organization is responsible for approving drugs, biologicals,
and medical devices and developing and enforcing food and drug
regulations.

Vaccine Knowledge Project
Centre for Clinical Vaccinology and Tropical Medicine
Churchill Hospital
University of Oxford, OX3 7LE
United Kingdom
http://vk.ovg.ox.ac.uk

The Vaccine Page
editor@vaccines.org
http://www.vaccines.org
A gateway site for up-to-the-minute vaccine news along with an an-
notated database of vaccine resource website. The site is supported by
vaccine advocacy groups such as the Allied Vaccine Group.

Wellcome Trust
Gibbs Building
215 Euston Road
London NW1 2BE
United Kingdom
44-(0)22-7611-8888
https://wellcome.ac.uk
The Wellcome Trust is a major partner in supporting vaccination programs in the United Kingdom and internationally through research
and outreach programs.

World Health Organization
20 Avenue Appia
1211 Geneva 27
Switzerland
http://www.who.int/topics/vaccines/en
The World Health Organization supports multiple international health initiatives, including an intensive immunization outreach and up-to-date information on vaccine research progress. Information is available in six languages.

ANTI-VACCINE AND VACCINE-SKEPTIC ORGANIZATIONS

Alliance for Human Research Protection
142 West End Ave., Suite 28P
New York, NY 10023
http://ahrp.org/category/s5-children/vaccine-safety

Australian Vaccination-Skeptics Network
PO Box 88
Bangalow, NSW 2479
Australia
https://avn.org.au
Australia's leading anti-vaccine organization provides information to counter mainstream scientific findings about vaccination.

Generation Rescue
13636 Ventura Blvd. #259
Sherman Oaks, CA 91423
877-98-AUTISM
http://www.generationrescue.org
Known as Jenny McCarthy's autism organization, this group provides autism information with an anti-vaccine slant and supports websites critiquing vaccine research.

National Vaccine Information Center
21525 Ridgetop Circle, Suite 100
Sterling, VA 20166
703-938-0342
contact@NVIC@gmail.com
https://www.nvic.org

A nonprofit organization cofounded in 1982 by vaccine skeptics Barbara Loe Fisher and Kathi Williams. The organization advocates for freedom of choice in vaccinating and vaccine safety with a vaccine-skeptic philosophy.

SafeMinds

10807 Falls Road, Suite 1416
Brooklandville, MD 21022
202-780-9821
https://safeminds.org
This autism advocacy organization has actively critiqued research suggesting there is no autism–vaccine link. It promotes risk-taking and experimental approaches to treating autism.

Vaccine Liberation

info@vaccinetruth.org
http://www.vaclib.org
This anti-vaccination organization has many state chapters and also provides information on foreign organizations that share its anti-vaccination views.

VaxTruth

www.vaxtruth.org
VaxTruth is an online anti-vaccination organization that provides information on vaccine ingredients, school exemptions from vaccination, and news articles about vaccines.

GLOSSARY

Adjuvant: A chemical added to a vaccine to boost immune response to an antigenic component.

Adverse effect: An undesirable, usually serious complication probably caused by the administration of a vaccine or a drug.

Adverse event: Any undesirable experience that occurs in a defined period after the administration of a vaccine or a drug. The vaccine or drug does not have to be the cause of the event.

Anaerobic: A bacterium that grows in the absence of oxygen (e.g., the bacterium that causes tetanus or botulism).

Anaphylaxis: A serious, life-threatening reaction. In hypersensitive individuals, anaphylaxis has causes as diverse as bee venom, peanuts, shellfish, and antigens in some vaccines.

Animal reservoir: Species of animals that can be infected by a virus that also infects humans so that the virus cannot be eradicated.

Antibody: A protein molecule (immunoglobulin) produced by B cells in response to a specific antigen.

Antibody titer test: A laboratory procedure for determining the strength of antibody production against an antigen.

Antigen: A nonself molecule that induces an immune system response, resulting in the production of antibodies.

Antigen-presenting cell: An immune system cell that engulfs a pathogen and then exhibits some of the pathogen's protein on its surface so that the antigen-presenting cell looks like a foreign cell. Macrophages and dendritic cells are the major antigen-presenting cells.

Attenuated: Said of a whole virus or bacterium that has been grown under adverse conditions or chemically treated so that it is weakened to the point where it does not cause the disease but stimulates an adequate immune response to it.

B cell: An antibody-producing cell that is part of the adaptive immune system.

Background rate: The frequency with which an adverse event occurs in an unvaccinated population. This rate is compared to the frequency of the same adverse event in a comparable vaccinated population to help determine if the vaccine causes an increase in occurrence of the adverse event.

Biologic product: A medical product made from natural sources such as human or animal cells, or microorganisms.

Blood serum: The clear yellowish fluid that remains after blood cells and clotting factors have been removed from whole blood.

Bone marrow: Soft tissue that fills the hollow spaces of bones. Red bone marrow produces stem cells that become erythrocytes (red blood cells), lymphocytes (white blood cells), and platelets. Yellow bone marrow produces stem cells that become fat, bone, and cartilage. Red and yellow bone marrow exist within the same bone cavities.

Clinical trial: A research study using humans in which volunteers are assigned to various groups to test the safety and effectiveness of a drug before it is licensed for public use.

Clonal expansion: The ability of a cell to divide and create millions of identical daughter cells.

Cold chain: A continuous system of cold boxes, refrigerators, and freezers used to keep biological products such as vaccines within a narrow temperature range during transport, distribution, and storage to prevent loss of potency of the product.

Cytokines: Small signaling proteins released by cells that control the behavior of other cells and help mediate the immune response.

Encephalitis: Acute swelling and inflammation of the brain that can result in permanent brain damage.

Formalin: A solution of formaldehyde and water.

Guillain-Barré syndrome (GBS): A rare syndrome in which the immune system attacks healthy nerve cells resulting in weakness or tingling sensations that move up the body and can cause paralysis. GBS appears to increase after infection with the Zika virus. There has been some controversy over whether influenza vaccination also increases the incidence of GBS.

Hematopoietic stem cells: Stem cells in the bone marrow that have the potential to differentiate into many different types of blood cells.

Herd immunity: Also called community immunity, this condition occurs when a high-enough percentage of the population is immune to a contagious disease through vaccination or naturally acquired immunity that there is little opportunity for the disease to spread to nonimmune individuals.

Immune tolerance: The ability of the immune system to recognize and leave unharmed an individual's self cells while attacking foreign cells and material.

Immunity: In medicine, the ability of an organism to resist disease, usually through the development of antibodies against the disease-causing pathogen. In law, exemption from certain legal proceedings, such as being sued or prosecuted for a crime.

Immunocompromised: Having a weakened immune system. Most common causes are chemotherapy, radiation therapy, steroid drugs, HIV infection, and inherited immune system disorders.

Immunological memory: The ability of T and B cells in the adaptive immune system to recognize a previously encountered pathogen and rapidly activate a defense against it so that the individual does not become sick.

Leukocytes: White blood cells.

Lymph: A clear, yellowish liquid that contains white blood cells. It flows through lymphatic vessels and is eventually returned to the circulatory system.

Lymph nodes: Also called lymph glands. Small bean-shaped organs located in the lymphatic system that filter out foreign pathogens. In humans, they are most prominent in the neck, armpits, and groin.

Major histocompatibility complex: A set of molecules on the surface of a cell that identify it as a self cell or a foreign cell. In humans, these molecules are also called human leukocyte antigens.

Memory cell: A long-lived lymphocyte that has encountered an antigen and on re-encountering it can initiate a rapid immune response (T memory cell) or make antibodies against the antigen (B memory cell).

Natural selection: A process by which organisms best suited to the environment survive and produce more offspring, whereas organisms that are less well adapted to the environment have reduced reproductive capacity or die.

Nucleus: A distinct organelle that contains genetic material (DNA) found in the cytoplasm of the cell. Most cells have a nucleus, although mature human red blood cells (erythrocytes) do not.

Peer review: A prepublication process used by journals that publish the results of scientific research. It involves sending the manuscript under consideration to several experts in the field who evaluate the importance of the study, the study's design, and the appropriateness of the data analysis to determine if the material is reliable enough to be published.

Peyer's patches: Small areas of lymphoid tissue found in the wall of the small intestine that promote the development of immunity to antigens found in the gut.

Placebo: A harmless substance given to some volunteers during clinical trials so that their responses can be compared to the volunteers who are given the trial drug or vaccine.

Plasma cell: A specialized cell of the adaptive immune system that produces antibodies.

Preservative: An antiseptic chemical used to kill bacteria and fungi that could contaminate a vaccine.

Primary response: The time it takes for the immune system to make enough antibodies against a pathogen to control a disease the first time the pathogen is encountered, usually 10–17 days.

Ring vaccination: A method of evaluating the effectiveness of a vaccine by vaccinating all the people exposed to an infected individual and determining how many become sick.

Secondary response: Stimulation of antibody production by memory cells on re-encountering a pathogen, usually taking two to seven days. Rapid secondary response is the basis for active immunity.

Spleen: The largest lymphoid organ in the body. Located to the left of the stomach and below the diaphragm, it produces lymphocytes (white blood cells) and removes old and damaged red blood cells from the blood.

Stabilizer: Substance added to a vaccine to shield it against temperature changes and to maintain its potency and extend its shelf life.

Subunit vaccine: A vaccine made by identifying and isolating the pathogen's antigenic proteins without including any of the pathogen's genetic material.

T cell: One of several related cells that mature in the thymus and help direct the chain of reactions that result in adaptive immunity.

Thymus: A butterfly-shaped lymphatic organ essential to the production of T cells. It gradually decreases in size after puberty.

Vector: An organism, often a biting insect or tick, that transmits a disease from one animal to another or from an infected animal to a human.

Zoonoses: Diseases that normally exist in animals but that can be transmitted to humans and cause illness.

BIBLIOGRAPHY

Age of Autism. "Transcript: Statement from Andrew Wakefield." April 13, 2017. www.ageofautism.com/2013/04/transcript-statement-from-andrew-wakefield .html (accessed September 5, 2018).

Ashland Child. "Alternative Schedule." AshlandChild.org 2018. https://www.ash landchild.org/vaccine-basics/alternative-schedule (accessed March 4, 2018).

Autism Speaks. "Policy Statement on Mercury and Autism." 2018. https://www .autismspeaks.org/about-us/press-releases/policy-statement-mercury-and-autism (accessed April 13, 2018).

Baker, Jeffrey. "Mercury, Vaccines, and Autism: One Controversy, Three Histories." *American Journal of Public Health* 98, no. 2 (February 2008): 244–253. https://www.ncbi.nlm.nih.gov/pmc/articles/PMC2376879 (accessed February 26, 2018).

Barrett, Stephen. "Chiropractors and Immunization." *Chirobase.* March 10, 2015. https://www.chirobase.org/06DD/chiroimmu.html (accessed September 5, 2017).

Beck, Ann. "Issues in the Anti-Vaccination Movement in England." *Medical History* 4, no. 4 (October 1960): 310–321. https://www.ncbi.nlm.nih.gov/pmc/ articles/PMC1034558 (accessed September 18, 2017).

Blaskiewicz, Robert. "The Big Pharma Conspiracy Theory." *Medical Writing* 22, no. 4 (2013): 259–261. journal.emwa.org/good-pharma/the-big-pharma-conspiracy-theory (accessed March 8, 2018).

Case, Brad. *Thugs, Drugs, and the War on Bugs: How the Natural Healthcare Revolution Will Lead Us Past Greed, Ego, and Scary Germs.* Prunedale, CA: New Renaissance Books, 2010.

College of Physicians of Philadelphia. "Misconceptions about Vaccines." 2018. https://www.historyofvaccines.org/content/articles/misconceptions-about-vaccines (accessed April 29, 2018).

Conte, Louis, and Tony Lyons. *Vaccine Injuries: Documented Adverse Reactions to Vaccines,* 2014–2015 edition. New York: Skyhorse Publishing, 2014.

Croston, Glenn E. *The Real Story of Risk: Adventures in a Hazardous World.* Amherst, NY: Prometheus Books, 2012.

Curtis, Tom. "The Origin of Aids: A Startling New Theory Attempts to Answer the Question 'Was It an Act of God or an Act of Man?'" *Rolling Stone* 626 (March 19, 1992): 54–59, 61, 106, 108. https://www.uow.edu.au/~bmartin/dissent/documents/AIDS/Curtis92.html (accessed May 2, 2018).

Davidson, Tish. *Vaccines: History, Science, and Issues.* Santa Barbara, CA: Greenwood Press, 2017.

Deer, Brian. "Exposed: Andrew Wakefield and the MMR-Autism Fraud." Brian Deer.com. http://briandeer.com/mmr/lancet-summary.htm (accessed September 16, 2017).

Deer, Brian. "Wakefield Filed for a Patent on Vaccine Products before Unleashing MMR Crisis." *BrianDeer.com.* http://briandeer.com/wakefield/wakefield-patents.htm (accessed May 2, 2018).

Dubé, Eve, Maryline Vivion, and Noni E. MacDonald. "Vaccine Hesitancy, Vaccine Refusal and the Anti-Vaccine Movement: Influence, Impact, and Implications." *Expert Reviews Vaccines* 14, no. 1 (2015): 99–117.

Earl, Elizabeth. "The Victorian Anti-Vaccination Movement." *The Atlantic.* July 15, 2015. https://www.theatlantic.com/health/archive/2015/07/victorian-anti-vaccinators-personal-belief-exemption/398321 (accessed August 6, 2018).

England, Christine. "Vaccines Have Destroyed Lives for Decades and the UK Government Tried to Cover It Up." Vactruth.com. June 16, 2010. https://vactruth.com/2010/06/16/vaccines-have-destroyed-lives-for-decades-and-the-uk-government-tried-to-cover-it-up (accessed August 6, 2018).

Espejo, Roman. *Should Vaccines Be Mandatory? (At Issue).* Farmington Hills, MI: Greenhaven Press, 2014.

Feemster, Kristen A. "Vaccine Hesitancy and Alternative Vaccine Schedules." Webinar. April 21, 2016. VaccineHesitancyFeemster4–21–16.pdf (accessed March 7, 2018).

Feemster, Kristen A. *Vaccines: What Everyone Needs to Know.* Oxford, UK; New York: Oxford University Press, 2018.

Fox, Rosemary. *Helen's Story.* London: John Blake, 2006.

Frompovich, Catherine J. "Vaccine Maker Admits on FDA Website That DTaP Vaccine Causes Autism." Activist Post: Alternative News & Independent Views. April 1, 2016. https://www.activistpost.com/2016/04/vaccine-maker-admits-on-fda-website-dtap-vaccine-causes-autism.html (accessed February 9, 2018).

Gladen, Eric. *Trace Amounts.* FAZE Films, 2014.

Gleberzon, Brian. "On Vaccination & Chiropractic: When Ideology, History, Perception, Politics, and Jurisprudence Collide." *Journal of the Canadian Chiropractic Association* 57, no. 3 (September 2013): 205–213. https://www.ncbi.nlm.nih.gov/pmc/articles/PMC3743646 (accessed January 24, 2018).

Gowada, Charitha, and Amanda F. Dempsey. "The Rise (and Fall?) of Parental Vaccine Hesitancy." *Human Vaccines & Immunotherapeutics* 9, no. 8 (2013): 1755–1762.

Habakus, Louise Kou, and Mary Holland, eds. *Vaccine Epidemic: How Corporate Greed, Biased Science, and Coercive Government Threaten Our Human Rights, Our Health, and Our Children.* New York: Skyhorse Publishing, 2011.

Haelle, Tara. "Pediatrician Bob Sears Punished for Questionable Vaccine Exemption." *Forbes* July 1, 2018. https://www.forbes.com/sites/tarahaelle/2018/07/01/pediatrician-bob-sears-license-temporarily-revoked-after-questionable-vaccine-exemption/#4df68026ef60 (accessed August 6, 2018).

Health Resources and Services Administration. "What You Need to Know about the Vaccine Injury Compensation Program (VICP)." September 2016. https://www.hrsa.gov/vaccine-compensation/index.html (accessed April 24, 2018).

Hilts, Donna. "TV Report on Vaccine Stirs Bitter Controversy." *Washington Post.* April 28, 1982. https://www.washingtonpost.com/archive/local/1982/04/28/tv-report-on-vaccine-stirs-bitter-controversy/80d1fc8a-1012-4732-a517-7976c86ab52d/?utm_term=.bb40d54a99b5 (accessed May 2, 2018).

Hornsey, M. J., E. A. Harris, and K. S. Fielding. "The Psychological Roots of Anti-Vaccination Attitudes: A 24-Nation Investigation." *Health Psychology* (February 1, 2018). Advance online publication. http://dx.doi.org/10.1037/hea0000586 (accessed March 8, 2018).

Horwin, Michael. "Simian Virus 40 (SV40): A Cancer Causing Monkey Virus from FDA-Approved Vaccines." *Albany Law Journal of Science & Technology* 13 no. 3 (2003): xx. http://www.sv40foundation.org/cpv-link.html (accessed May 2, 2018).

International Foundation for Nutrition and Health. "Dr. Henry. G. Bieler." http://ifnh.org/dr-henry-g-bieler (accessed August 6, 2018).

Institute of Medicine (US) Immunization Safety Review Committee. "Immunization Safety Review: Vaccines and Autism." Washington, DC: National Academy of Sciences Press, 2004. https://www.ncbi.nlm.nih.gov/pubmed/20669467 (accessed February 28, 2018).

Jaffe, Rick. "Dr. Bob Sears Medical Board Case Update: LA Times Tries to Squeeze, Shame and Goad the California Medical Board to Go after Bob Sears and Other Vaccine Exemption Writing Docs Harder and Faster." Blog Post. November 6, 2017. http://rickjaffeesq.com/2017/11/06/dr-bob-sears-medical-board-case-update-la-times-tries-squeeze-shame-goad-california-medical-board-go-bob-sears-vaccine-exemption-writing-docs-harder-faster (accessed March 8, 2018).

Karlamangla, Soumya. "Opponents Sue to Stop California's Vaccination Law." *Los Angeles Times.* July 5, 2016. http://www.latimes.com/local/lanow/la-me-ln-vaccination-lawsuit-20160705-snap-story.html (accessed March 1, 2018).

Karlamangla, Soumya, and Rong-Gong Lin II. "Vaccination Rate Jumps in California after Tougher Inoculation Law." *Los Angeles Times.* April 13, 2017. http://www.latimes.com/local/lanow/la-me-ln-california-vaccination-20170412-story.html (accessed May 2, 2018).

Kata, Anna. "Anti-Vaccine Activists, Web 2.0, and the Postmodern Paradigm—
    An Overview of Tactics and Tropes Used Online by the Anti-Vaccination
    Movement." *Vaccine* 30 (2012): 3778–3789.
Kata, Anna. "A Postmodern Pandora's Box: Anti-Vaccination Misinformation on
    the Internet." *Vaccine* 20 (2010): 1709–1716.
Kennedy, Robert F., Jr. "Mercury Is Not Safe in Any Form: Debunking the Myths
    about Thimerosal 'Safety.'" World Mercury Project 2016. https://world
    mercuryproject.org/thimerosal-history/mercury-is-not-safe-in-any-form-
    debunking-the-myths-about-thimerosal-safety (accessed April 13, 2018).
Kennedy, Robert F., Jr. *Thimerosal: Let Science Speak*. New York: Skyhorse Pub-
    lishing, 2014.
Kennedy, Robert F., Jr. "Yale University Study Shows Association between Vac-
    cines and Brain Disorders." EcoWatch. February 8, 2017. https://www.ecow
    atch.com/yale-vaccine-study-kennedy-2246059411.html (accessed Febru-
    ary 11, 2018).
Kestenbaum, Lori, and Kristen A. Feemster. "Identifying and Addressing Vac-
    cine Hesitancy." *Pediatric Annals* 44 no. 4 (April 2015): e71–e75. https://
    www.ncbi.nlm.nih.gov/pmc/articles/PMC4475845 (accessed September 17,
    2017).
Kirby, David. *Evidence of Harm: Mercury in Vaccines and the Autism Epidemic:
    A Medical Controversy*. New York: St. Martin's Press, 2005.
Kluger, Jeffrey. "Jim Carrey, Please Shut Up about Vaccines." *Time*. July 2,
    2015. http://time.com/3944067/jim-carrey-vaccines (accessed February 2,
    2018).
Krishnan, Shobha S. *The HPV Vaccine Controversy: Sex, Cancer, God, and Poli-
    tics: A Guide for Parents, Women, Men, and Teenagers*. Westport, CT: Prae-
    ger, 2008.
Lam, Bourree. "Vaccines Are Profitable, So What?" *The Atlantic*. February 10,
    2015. https://www.theatlantic.com/business/archive/2015/02/vaccines-are-
    profitable-so-what/385214 (accessed March 8, 2018).
Largent, Mark A. *Vaccine: The Debate in Modern America*. Baltimore: Johns
    Hopkins University Press, 2012.
Leslie, Douglas L., et al. "Temporal Association of Certain Neuropsychiatric Dis-
    orders Following Vaccination of Children and Adolescents: A Pilot Case—
    Control Study." *Frontiers in Psychiatry*. January 19, 2017. https://www
    .frontiersin.org/articles/10.3389/fpsyt.2017.00003/full (accessed February 9,
    2018).
McNeil, Donald G., Jr. "Flu Patients Arrive in Droves, and a Hospital Rolls Out
    the 'Surge Tent.'" *New York Times*. February 2, 2018. https://www.nytimes
    .com/2018/02/02/health/flu-symptoms-virus-hospital.html (accessed March 8,
    2018).
Merino, Noel. *Vaccines. (At Issue)*. Farmington Hills, MI: Greenhaven Press,
    2015.
Mnookin, Seth. *The Panic Virus*. New York: Simon & Schuster, 2011.
National Center for Health Statistics. "Immunization." 2017. https://www.cdc
    .gov/nchs/fastats/immunize.htm (accessed March 28, 2017).

Offit, Paul A. (MD). *Deadly Choices: How the Anti-Vaccine Movement Threatens Us All*. New York: Basic Books, 2011.

Offit, Paul, and Charlotte Moser. "The Problem with Dr. Bob's Alternative Vaccine Schedule." *Pediatrics* 123 no. 1 (January 2009): e164–e169. http://pedi atrics.aappublications.org/content/123/1/e164 (accessed March 2, 2018).

"Origin of AIDS Update." *Rolling Stone*. December 9, 1993, p. 39. https://www .uow.edu.au/~bmartin/dissent/documents/AIDS/rs93.html (accessed May 2, 2018).

Oster, Emily, and Geoffrey Kocks. "After a Debacle, How California Became a Model on Measles." *New York Times*. January 16, 2018. https://www.nytimes .com/2018/01/16/upshot/measles-vaccination-california-students.html?_r=0 (accessed January 18, 2018.)

Palmer, Bartlett Joshua. *The Philosophy of Chiropractic*. Davenport, IA: Palmer School of Chiropractic Publishing, 1909.

Palmer, David D. *The Chiropractor's Adjustor*. Portland, OR: Portland Printing House Company, 1910.

Plotkin, Stanley, Jeffrey S. Gerber, and Paul Offit. "Vaccines and Autism: A Tale of Shifting Hypotheses." *Clinical Infectious Diseases* 48, no. 4 (February 15, 2009): 456–461. https://academic.oup.com/cid/article/48/4/456/284219 (accessed February 28, 2018).

Polio Global Eradication Initiative. "This Week." 2018. http://polioeradication .org/polio-today/polio-now/this-week (accessed April 28, 2018).

ProCon.org. "State Vaccinations Exemptions for Children Entering Public Schools." July 8, 2016. http://vaccines.procon.org/view.resource.php?resource ID=003597 (accessed April 29, 2018).

Public Broadcasting System. "The Vaccine War." *Frontline*. April 10, 2010. http:// www.pbs.org/video/frontline-vaccine-war (accessed March 5, 2018).

Public Broadcasting System. *Frontline*. "Jenny McCarthy: 'We're Not an Anti-Vaccine Movement . . . We're Pro-Safe Vaccine.'" March 23, 2015. Transcript. https://www.pbs.org/wgbh/frontline/article/jenny-mccarthy-were-not-an-anti-vaccine-movement-were-pro-safe-vaccine (accessed January 31, 2018).

Public Broadcasting System. *Nova*. 2014. Transcript. http://www.pbs.org/wgbh/ nova/body/vaccines-calling-shots.html (accessed February 7, 2018).

Quakenboss, Levi. "Why Is the Media Attacking the Flu Vaccine?" Blog Post. September 14, 2017. https://leviquackenboss.wordpress.com/2017/09/14/ why-is-the-media-attacking-the-flu-vaccine (accessed March 8, 2018).

Reiss, Dorit Rubinstein. "Index of Articles by Dorit Rubenstein Reiss." January 2015. *Skeptical Raptor*. http://www.skepticalraptor.com/skepticalraptorblog .php/index-articles-guest-author-professor-dorit-rubinstein-reiss (accessed April 29, 2018).

Rhode, Wayne. *The Vaccine Court: The Dark Truth of America's Vaccine Injury Compensation Program*. New York: Skyhorse Publishing, 2014.

Ruishalme, Iida. "Myth: No Studies Compare the Health of Unvaccinated and Vaccinated People." *Thoughtscapism*. April 10, 2015. https://thoughtscap ism.com/2015/04/10/myth-no-studies-compare-the-health-of-unvaccinated-and-vaccinated-people (accessed February 1, 2018).

Sadaf, Alina, et al. "A Systematic Review of Interventions for Reducing Parental Vaccine Refusal and Vaccine Hesitancy." *Vaccine* 31 (2013): 4293–4304.

SanofiPasteur. "Diphtheria and Tetanus Toxoids and Acellular Pertussis Vaccine Adsorbed" [FDA Package Insert]. December 2005. https://vaccines.procon .org/sourcefiles/DTaP_Tripedia.pdf (accessed February 9, 2018).

Scheibner, Viera. "History and Science Show That Vaccines Do Not Prevent Disease." *Health Impact News*. 2013. http://healthimpactnews.com/2013/ history-and-science-show-vaccines-do-not-prevent-disease (accessed September 16, 2017).

Scutti, Susan. "How Countries around the World Try to Encourage Vaccination." CNN.com. January 2, 2018. https://www.cnn.com/2017/06/06/health/vac cine-uptake-incentives/index.html (accessed March 1, 2018).

Sears, Robert. *The Vaccine Book: Making the Right Decision for Your Child*, 2nd ed. New York: Little, Brown, 2011.

Sharav, Vera. "L'affaire Wakefield: Shades of Dreyfus & BMJ's Descent into Tabloid Science." Alliance for Human Research Protection. October 30, 2017. http://ahrp.org/laffaire-wakefield-shades-of-dreyfus-bmjs-descent-into-tab loid-science (accessed February 21, 2018).

Shaw, George Bernard. "Mr. Bernard Shaw on Vaccination." *British Medical Journal* 2, no. 2181 (October 16, 1901): 1283. https://www.ncbi.nlm.nih .gov/pmc/articles/PMC2401975/?page=1 G. Bernard Shaw (accessed May 2, 2018).

Snopes.com. "Is Autism Now Disclosed as a DTaP Vaccine Side Effect?" Snopes .com. November 20, 2017. https://www.snopes.com/autism-is-now-disclosed-as-dtap-side-effect (accessed February 9, 2018).

Sohn, Emily. "Understanding the History behind Communities' Vaccine Fears." National Public Radio. May 3, 2017. https://www.npr.org/sections/health-shots/2017/05/03/526595475/understanding-the-history-behind-communi ties-vaccine-fears (accessed April 28, 2018).

Stein, Richard. "The Golden Age of Anti-Vaccine Conspiracies." *Germs* 7, no. 4 (December 2017): 168–170. https://www.ncbi.nlm.nih.gov/pmc/articles/ PMC5734925 (accessed March 8, 2018).

Thomas, Paul, and Jennifer Margulis. *The Vaccine-Friendly Plan*. New York: Ballantine Books, 2016.

Thompson, William. "A Bad Day for Anti-Vaccinationists: A Possible Retraction, and the 'CDC Whistleblower' William W. Thompson Issues a Statement." August 28, 2014. https://respectfulinsolence.com/2014/08/28/a-bad-day-for-antivaccinationists-a-retraction-and-the-cdc-whistleblower-issues-a-state ment (accessed March 9, 2018).

UK Patent Application GB 2 325 856 A. http://briandeer.com/wakefield/wake field-patents.htm (accessed May 1, 2018).

United States Centers for Disease Control and Prevention. "The Pink Book." 2016. https://www.cdc.gov/vaccines/pubs/pinkbook/chapters.html (accessed September 26, 2017).

United States Centers for Disease Control and Prevention. "Recommended Immunization Schedule for Children and Adolescents Aged 18 Years or Younger, United States, 2018." https://www.cdc.gov/vaccines/schedules/hcp/imz/child-adolescent.html (accessed March 6, 2018).

United States Centers for Disease Control and Protection. "Science Summary: CDC Studies on Thimerosal in Vaccines." 2013. https://www.cdc.gov/vaccinesafety/pdf/cdcstudiesonvaccinesandautism.pdf (accessed February 28, 2018).

United States District Court for the Eastern District of Virginia (Alexandria Division) Barbara Loe Arthur (AKA Barbara Loe Fisher) v. Paul Offit, M.D., Amy Wallace, and Condé Nast Publishers. Complaint with Demand for Jury Trial. Dismissed February 3, 2010. https://www.nivc.org/cmstemplates.nvic/pdf/offit-wired/blf-vs-offit-plaintifs-opposition-to-defendant.pdf (accessed April 28, 2018).

United States Food and Drug Administration. "Thimerosal in Vaccines." May 16, 2017. https://www.fda.gov/BiologicsBloodVaccines/SafetyAvailability/VaccineSafety/UCM096228 (accessed September 12, 2017).

United States Senate Committee on Health, Education, Labor, and Pensions. "Executive Summary of the Report of the Ranking Member on Alleged Misconduct by Government Agencies and Private Entities Related to Thimerosal in Childhood Vaccines." September 2007. https://vaccines.procon.org/sourcefiles/Thimerosal_and_ASD_Enzi_Report.pdf (accessed May 2, 2018).

United States Senate Committee on Health, Education, Labor, and Pensions. "Thimerosal and Autism Spectrum Disorders: Alleged Misconduct by Government Agencies and Private Entities." September 2007. Thimerosal_and_ASD_Enzi_Report.pdf (accessed April 9, 2018).

Vaccine Education Center. "Aluminium in Vaccines: What You Should Know." V.5, Winter 2014. media.chop.edu/data/files/pdfs/vaccine-education-center-aluminum.pdf (accessed February 1, 2018).

Vaccine Information Coalition. "Now It's Official: FDA Announced That Vaccines Are Causing Autism!" [undated]. http://www.vacinfo.org (accessed February 9, 2018).

"Vaccines Did Not Save Us." ChildHealthSafety.org. 2009. https://childhealthsafety.wordpress.com/graphs (accessed January 26, 2018).

Wakefield, Andrew. *Callous Disregard: Autism and Vaccines—The Truth behind a Tragedy*. New York: Skyhorse Pub., 2010.

Wakefield, Andrew. *Vaxxed: From Cover-Up to Catastrophe*. (DVD). Burbank, CA: Cinema Libra Studio, 2016.

Wakefield, Andrew, et al. "Ileal-Lymphoid-Nodular Hyperplasia, Non-Specific Colitis, and Pervasive Developmental Disorder in Children." *The Lancet* 351, no. 9103 (February 28, 1998): 637–641. Article Retracted 2004. http://www.thelancet.com/journals/lancet/article/PIIS0140-6736(97)11096-0/abstract (accessed April 6, 2018).

Wells, Jamie. "Debunking Vaccine Myths with Dr. Paul Offit." Transcript of American Council on Health and Science video. October 7, 2016. https://www .acsh.org/news/2016/10/07/debunking-vaccine-myths-dr-paul-offit-10269 (accessed February 1, 2018).

Wheeling, Kate. "A Brief History of Vaccine Conspiracy Theories." *Pacific Standard.* January 12, 2017. https://psmag.com/news/a-brief-history-of-vaccine-conspiracy-theories (accessed September 18, 2017).

Wolfe, Robert M., and Lisa K. Sharp. "Anti-Vaccinationists Past and Present." *British Medical Journal* 325 no. 7361 (August 24, 2002): 430–432.

World Health Organization. "Six Common Misconceptions about Immunization." 2018. http://www.who.int/vaccine_safety/initiative/detection/immunization_misconceptions/en/index1.html (accessed January 26, 2018)

World Health Organization. "Vaccine Safety Basics." 2017. http://vaccine-safety-training.org/Importance-of-immunization-programmes.html (accessed March 28, 2017).

Ziv, Stav. "Andrew Wakefield, Father of the Anti-Vaccine Movement, Responds to the Current Measles Outbreak for the First Time." *Newsweek.* February 10, 2015. http://www.newsweek.com/2015/02/20/andrew-wakefield-father-anti-vaccine-movement-sticks-his-story-305836.html (accessed February 21, 2018).

INDEX

About the Author

Tish Davidson, AM, is a medical writer specializing in making technical information accessible to general readership. She is the author of *Vaccines: History, Science, and Issues* and *Fluids and Electrolytes*, as well as contributor to *Biology: A Text for High School Students* and *Adolescent Health & Wellness*. Davidson holds membership in the American Medical Writers Association and the American Society of Journalists and Authors.